Exploring Novel Clinical Trial Designs for Gene-Based Therapies

PROCEEDINGS OF A WORKSHOP

Siobhan Addie, Meredith Hackmann, Joe Alper, and Sarah H. Beachy,
Rapporteurs

Forum on Regenerative Medicine

Board on Health Sciences Policy

Health and Medicine Division

The National Academies of
SCIENCES · ENGINEERING · MEDICINE

THE NATIONAL ACADEMIES PRESS
Washington, DC
www.nap.edu

THE NATIONAL ACADEMIES PRESS   500 Fifth Street, NW   Washington, DC 20001

This activity was supported by contracts between the National Academy of Sciences and Advanced Regenerative Manufacturing Institute; Akron Biotech; Alliance for Regenerative Medicine; American Society of Gene & Cell Therapy; Burroughs Wellcome Fund; California Institute for Regenerative Medicine; Centre for Commercialization of Regenerative Medicine; Department of Veterans Affairs (Contract No. VA268-16-C-0051); Food and Drug Administration (Grant #1R13FD0066—14-01); GE Healthcare; International Society for Cell & Gene Therapy; International Society for Stem Cell Research; Johnson & Johnson; The Michael J. Fox Foundation for Parkinson's Research; National Institute of Standards and Technology; National Institutes of Health: National Institute of Dental and Craniofacial Research (Contract No. HHSN263201800029I; Order No. 75N98019F00847), National Institute of Diabetes and Digestive and Kidney Diseases (PO No. 75N94019P00304); The New York Stem Cell Foundation; Parkinson's Foundation; Sanofi (Contract No. 55630791); and United Therapeutics Corporation (Contract No. 10003921). Any opinions, findings, conclusions, or recommendations expressed in this publication do not necessarily reflect the views of any organization or agency that provided support for the project.

International Standard Book Number-13: 978-0-309-67298-6
International Standard Book Number-10: 0-309-67298-8
Digital Object Identifier: http://doi.org/10.17226/25712

Additional copies of this publication are available from the National Academies Press, 500 Fifth Street, NW, Keck 360, Washington, DC 20001; (800) 624-6242 or (202) 334-3313; http://www.nap.edu.

Suggested citation: National Academies of Sciences, Engineering, and Medicine. 2020. *Exploring novel clinical trial designs for gene-based therapies: Proceedings of a workshop*. Washington, DC: The National Academies Press. http://doi. org/10.17226/25712.

The National Academies of
SCIENCES · ENGINEERING · MEDICINE

The National Academies of
SCIENCES · ENGINEERING · MEDICINE

PLANNING COMMITTEE ON EXPLORING NOVEL CLINICAL TRIAL DESIGNS FOR GENE-BASED THERAPIES[1]

KRISHANU SAHA (*Co-Chair*), Associate Professor and Retina Research Foundation Kathryn and Latimer Murfee Chair, Department of Biomedical Engineering, University of Wisconsin–Madison
CELIA WITTEN (*Co-Chair*), Deputy Director, Center for Biologics Evaluation and Research, Food and Drug Administration
MILDRED CHO, Research Professor of Pediatrics and Associate Director, Center for Biomedical Ethics, Stanford University
MICHAEL DeBAUN, Professor of Pediatrics and Medicine, Vanderbilt University School of Medicine
CYNTHIA DUNBAR, Senior Investigator, National Heart, Lung, and Blood Institute, National Institutes of Health
DEREK ROBERTSON, Co-Founder and President, Maryland Sickle Cell Disease Association
KATHERINE TSOKAS, Regulatory Head of Regenerative Medicine and Advanced Therapy, Johnson & Johnson

Forum on Regenerative Medicine Staff

SARAH H. BEACHY, Senior Program Officer and Forum Director
SIOBHAN ADDIE, Program Officer
MEREDITH HACKMANN, Associate Program Officer
MICHAEL BERRIOS, Senior Program Assistant

Board on Health Sciences Policy Staff

BRIDGET BOREL, Program Coordinator (*from October 2019*)
MARIAM SHELTON, Program Coordinator (*until October 2019*)
ANDREW M. POPE, Senior Board Director

---

[1] The National Academies of Sciences, Engineering, and Medicine's planning committees are solely responsible for organizing the workshop, identifying topics, and choosing speakers. The responsibility for the published proceedings of a workshop rests with the workshop rapporteurs and the institution.

FORUM ON REGENERATIVE MEDICINE[1]

TIM COETZEE (*Co-Chair*), Chief Advocacy, Services and Research Officer, National Multiple Sclerosis Society

KATHERINE TSOKAS (*Co-Chair*), Regulatory Head of Regenerative Medicine and Advanced Therapy, Johnson & Johnson

JAMES C. BECK, Vice President, Scientific Affairs, Parkinson's Foundation

SANGEETA BHATIA, John J. and Dorothy Wilson Professor, Institute for Medical Engineering and Science, Electrical Engineering and Computer Science, Massachusetts Institute of Technology

GEORGE Q. DALEY, Director, Stem Cell Transplantation Program, Boston Children's Hospital and Dana-Farber Cancer Institute; Dean, Harvard Medical School

BRIAN FISKE, Senior Vice President, Research Programs, The Michael J. Fox Foundation for Parkinson's Research

LAWRENCE GOLDSTEIN, Distinguished Professor, Department of Cellular and Molecular Medicine, Department of Neurosciences; Director, University of California, San Diego, Stem Cell Program; Scientific Director, Sanford Consortium for Regenerative Medicine; Director, Sanford Stem Cell Clinical Center, University of California, San Diego, School of Medicine

AUDREY KUSIAK, Scientific Program Manager, Rehabilitation Research and Development Service, Office of Research and Development, Department of Veterans Affairs (*until September 2019*)

ROBERT S. LANGER, David H. Koch Institute Professor, Massachusetts Institute of Technology

CATO T. LAURENCIN, University Professor, Albert and Wilda Van Dusen Distinguished Professor of Orthopaedic Surgery, Professor of Chemical, Materials Science, and Biomedical Engineering; Director, The Raymond and Beverly Sackler Center for Biomedical, Biological, Physical, and Engineering Sciences; Chief Executive Officer, Connecticut Convergence Institute for Translation in Regenerative Engineering, University of Connecticut

TERRY MAGNUSON, Sarah Graham Kenan Professor, Vice Chancellor for Research, University of North Carolina at Chapel Hill

MICHAEL MAY, President and Chief Executive Officer, Centre for Commercialization of Regenerative Medicine

---

[1]The National Academies of Sciences, Engineering, and Medicine's forums and roundtables do not issue, review, or approve individual documents. The responsibility for the published proceedings of a workshop rests with the workshop rapporteurs and the institution.

RICHARD McFARLAND, Chief Regulatory Officer, Advanced Regenerative Manufacturing Institute

JACK MOSHER, Senior Manager, Scientific Affairs, International Society for Stem Cell Research

DUANQING PEI, Director General, Guangzhou Institutes of Biomedicine and Health, Chinese Academy of Sciences

THOMAS PETERSEN, Vice President, Regenerative Medicine, United Therapeutics Corporation

ANNE PLANT, Chief of the Biosystems and Biomaterials Division, National Institute of Standards and Technology

KIMBERLEE POTTER, Scientific Program Manager, Biomedical Laboratory R&D Service, Office of Research and Development, Department of Veterans Affairs (*from September 2019*)

DEREK ROBERTSON, Co-Founder and President, Maryland Sickle Cell Disease Association

GRIFFIN RODGERS, Director, National Institute of Diabetes and Digestive and Kidney Diseases, National Institutes of Health

KELLY ROSE, Program Officer, Burroughs Wellcome Fund

KRISHNENDU ROY, Robert A. Milton Chair and Professor in Biomedical Engineering; Technical Lead, National Cell Manufacturing Consortium; Director, Marcus Center for Therapeutic Cell Characterization and Manufacturing, Georgia Institute of Technology

KRISHANU SAHA, Associate Professor and Retina Research Foundation Kathryn and Latimer Murfee Chair, Department of Biomedical Engineering, University of Wisconsin–Madison

RACHEL SALZMAN, Society Officer, American Society of Gene & Cell Therapy

JAY P. SIEGEL, Chief Biotechnology Officer and Head, Scientific Strategy and Policy, Johnson & Johnson (*Retired*)

LANA SKIRBOLL, Vice President, Science Policy, Sanofi

MARTHA SOMERMAN, Director, National Institute of Dental and Craniofacial Research, National Institutes of Health

LISA STROVINK, Chief Strategy Officer, The New York Stem Cell Foundation

SOHEL TALIB, Associate Director of Therapeutics and Industry Alliance, California Institute for Regenerative Medicine

PHIL VANEK, General Manager, Cell Therapy Growth Strategy, GE Healthcare

DANIEL WEISS, Chief Scientific Officer, International Society for Cell & Gene Therapy

MICHAEL WERNER, Co-Founder and Senior Policy Counsel, Alliance for Regenerative Medicine

CELIA WITTEN, Deputy Director, Center for Biologics Evaluation and
Research, Food and Drug Administration
CLAUDIA ZYLBERBERG, Founder and Chief Executive Officer,
Akron Biotech

Forum on Regenerative Medicine Staff

SARAH H. BEACHY, Senior Program Officer and Forum Director
SIOBHAN ADDIE, Program Officer
MEREDITH HACKMANN, Associate Program Officer
MICHAEL BERRIOS, Senior Program Assistant

Board on Health Sciences Policy Staff

BRIDGET BOREL, Program Coordinator (*from October 2019*)
MARIAM SHELTON, Program Coordinator (*until October 2019*)
ANDREW M. POPE, Senior Board Director

Reviewers

This Proceedings of a Workshop was reviewed in draft form by individuals chosen for their diverse perspectives and technical expertise. The purpose of this independent review is to provide candid and critical comments that will assist the National Academies of Sciences, Engineering, and Medicine in making each published proceedings as sound as possible and to ensure that it meets the institutional standards for quality, objectivity, evidence, and responsiveness to the charge. The review comments and draft manuscript remain confidential to protect the integrity of the process.

We thank the following individuals for their review of this proceedings:

ALEXANDRA BEATTY, National Academies of Sciences,
    Engineering, and Medicine
ROSEMARIE HUNZIKER, Connexon Life Science Consulting
DEREK ROBERTSON, Maryland Sickle Cell Disease Association

Although the reviewers listed above provided many constructive comments and suggestions, they were not asked to endorse the content of the proceedings nor did they see the final draft before its release. The review of this proceedings was overseen by **LESLIE BENET,** University of California, San Francisco. He was responsible for making certain that an independent examination of this proceedings was carried out in accordance with standards of the National Academies and that all review comments were carefully considered. Responsibility for the final content rests entirely with the rapporteurs and the National Academies.

Acknowledgments

The support of the sponsors of the Forum on Regenerative Medicine was crucial to the planning and conduct of the workshop Exploring Novel Clinical Trial Designs for Gene-Based Therapies, and for the development of this Proceedings of a Workshop. Federal sponsors were the Department of Veterans Affairs; Food and Drug Administration; National Institute of Standards and Technology; and National Institutes of Health: National Institute of Dental and Craniofacial Research and National Institute of Diabetes and Digestive and Kidney Diseases. Nonfederal sponsorship was provided by the Advanced Regenerative Manufacturing Institute; Akron Biotech; Alliance for Regenerative Medicine; American Society of Gene & Cell Therapy; Burroughs Wellcome Fund; California Institute for Regenerative Medicine; Centre for Commercialization of Regenerative Medicine; GE Healthcare; International Society for Cell & Gene Therapy; International Society for Stem Cell Research; Johnson & Johnson; The Michael J. Fox Foundation for Parkinson's Research; The New York Stem Cell Foundation; Parkinson's Foundation; Sanofi; and United Therapeutics Corporation.

The Forum on Regenerative Medicine wishes to express gratitude to the expert speakers who explored the design complexities and ethical issues associated with developing clinical trials for gene-based therapies. The forum also wishes to thank the members of the planning committee for their work in developing an excellent workshop agenda. The project director would like to thank the project staff who worked diligently to develop both the workshop and the resulting Proceedings of a Workshop.

Contents

xv

Boxes, Figures, and Table

BOXES

FIGURES

TABLE

Acronyms and Abbreviations

AAV	adeno-associated virus
ADA	adenosine deaminase
BEST	Biomarkers, EndpointS, and other Tools
CAR T	chimeric antigen receptor T cell
CCSS	Childhood Cancer Survivor Study
CFTR	cystic fibrosis transmembrane conductance regulator
CLL	chronic lymphocytic leukemia
CNS	central nervous system
DDT	drug development tool
DMD	Duchenne muscular dystrophy
Dx	diagnosis
FDA	Food and Drug Administration
GAA	acid alpha-glucosidase
GT	gene therapy
GVHD	graft-versus-host disease
HL	Hodgkin lymphoma
HLA	human leukocyte antigen

IRB   institutional review board

MLMT   multi-luminance mobility test

NCATS   National Center for Advancing Translational Sciences
NCI   National Cancer Institute
NDI   National Death Index
NeuroNEXT   Network for Excellence in Neuroscience Clinical Trials
NHL   non-Hodgkin lymphoma
NHLBI   National Heart, Lung, and Blood Institute
NIH   National Institutes of Health

RPE65   retinal pigment epithelium 65

SCD   sickle cell disease
SCID   severe combined immunodeficiency
SJLIFE   St. Jude Lifetime cohort
SMA   spinal muscular atrophy

1

Introduction and Overview[1]

Gene therapy is a technique that uses or modifies genes to prevent or treat disease. Gene therapy approaches are diverse and can include replacing a disease-causing gene with a correct copy, inactivating a gene that is functioning improperly, and introducing a new gene into the body to help fight disease, among other approaches (NLM, 2020). At the time of this workshop, the Food and Drug Administration (FDA) had approved four gene therapy products for use, including two genetically modified T-cell immunotherapies for different types of leukemia and lymphoma, one gene therapy for patients with mutation-associated retinal dystrophy, and one gene therapy for children less than 2 years old with spinal muscular atrophy.[2] The design of clinical trials for gene therapy products is often complex and can present many translational, clinical, and ethical issues, including challenges with determining an optimal dosage, delivering the product effectively, and successfully recruiting patients and following them over the long term. Patients and clinicians may also face difficult decisions about enrolling in gene therapy trials because of uncertainty about

---

[1] The planning committee's role was limited to planning the workshop, and the Proceedings of a Workshop was prepared by the workshop rapporteurs as a factual summary of what occurred at the workshop. Statements, recommendations, and opinions expressed are those of individual presenters and participants, and are not necessarily endorsed or verified by the National Academies of Sciences, Engineering, and Medicine, and they should not be construed as reflecting any group consensus.

[2] See Approved Cellular and Gene Therapy Products at https://www.fda.gov/vaccines-blood-biologics/cellular-gene-therapy-products/approved-cellular-and-gene-therapy-products (accessed January 12, 2020).

potentially long-lasting effects and concerns related to the future use of other therapeutic options, including different gene therapies.

One challenge, for example, is selecting an appropriate study population for a first-in-human clinical trial with a gene therapy whose greatest potential for clinical benefits is in very young children. For such therapies, it is important to identify ways to balance the potential clinical benefits with available safety data and to address when it would be appropriate to rely on data obtained from the preclinical program and natural history studies to support administering novel gene therapies to young children.

Another type of challenge faces clinical trials with gene therapies aimed at treating or curing rare genetic diseases, as the number of patients who are eligible to receive an experimental therapy during a clinical trial may be very limited. To address this, finding approaches that enable the effective use of data collected in natural history studies can further improve the efficiency of developing the gene therapies.

Yet another challenging set of issues in gene therapy trials involves dose selection and considerations for the possibility of repeat gene therapy administration. Gene therapy products often have long-lasting activity, and their administration may result in the formation of neutralizing antibodies or induce a pathologic immune response. A subsequent product administration to the same patient may result in lack of efficacy or severe toxicity that may preclude a repeat administration of the same therapy or a different therapy that targets the same gene, cell type, or tissue, or uses the same vector. Recognizing and managing immunogenicity in clinical trials, determining the appropriate product dosing and administration, and carefully monitoring for long-term effects of gene therapies are important tactics to employ when developing these novel treatments.

Those in the field have also found it challenging to measure the treatment benefits of gene therapies accurately. Changes in the expression and levels of transgene proteins (e.g., enzymes, blood clotting factors) following the administration of a gene therapy may not always be predictive of clinical benefits. Gaining a thorough understanding of how to optimally evaluate the clinical meaningfulness of blood and tissue measurements of transgene protein and creating reliable, functional assays may result in improved trial endpoints. Lastly, a clear understanding of the disease mechanism(s) and progression can be important for quantifying the clinical effectiveness of a gene therapy.

The scientific and translational issues described above are accompanied by myriad ethical issues, such as fairness in the selection of patients for trial participation, informed consent, and benevolence on the part of health care providers administering the experimental gene therapies. Developing improved educational tools to help patients and their providers understand the potential risks and benefits of specific gene therapies may help the field move forward. Recognizing the potential design complexities and ethical issues associated with clinical trials for these types of therapies, the Forum on Regenerative Medicine held a 1-day workshop in Washington, DC, on November 13, 2019, to explore these issues with a variety of stakeholders in greater detail. Speakers at the workshop discussed patient recruitment and selection for gene-based clinical trials, explored how the safety of new therapies is assessed, reviewed the challenges involving dose escalation, and spoke about ethical issues such as informed consent and the role of clinicians in recommending trials as options to their patients. The workshop also included discussions of topics related to gene therapies in the context of other available and potentially curative treatments, such as bone marrow transplantation for hemoglobinopathies. The concept of repeat dosing and sensitization treatments was also explored by the broad array of stakeholders who took part in the workshop, including academic and industry researchers, regulatory officials, clinicians, bioethicists, individuals and patients, and representatives of patient advocacy groups. The workshop agenda is in Appendix A, biographical sketches of the speakers and moderators are in Appendix B, the Statement of Task for the workshop is in Appendix C, and the list of workshop attendees is in Appendix D.

In his introductory remarks to the workshop, Krishanu Saha, an associate professor and the Retina Research Foundation Kathryn and Latimer Murfee Chair in the Department of Biomedical Engineering at the University of Wisconsin–Madison, discussed the differences in how gene-based therapies move through clinical trials compared with most drugs in development. Typically, he explained, drug discovery and development entails screening thousands of compounds for the desired properties, conducting extensive preclinical studies, and enrolling hundreds if not thousands of patients in multiple clinical trials that can take 6 to 7 years to complete. From discovery to market, it is not uncommon for the drug development process to take 10 to 15 years (Janssen Pharmaceutica, 2020).

In contrast, gene-based therapy development starts with a few therapeutic candidates that developers test in 100 or fewer patients—or, in some cases, individual patients, Saha noted. In fact, the faces and names of these patients are often widely recognized and have been featured by major new outlets. The preclinical process, Saha said, which can take 3 to 6 years with traditional drug candidates, can be completed in 1 to 3 years with gene-based therapies. Another difference is that the therapeutic candidates themselves—cells, viruses, genome editors, antisense oligonucleotides, and others—are more complex than small-molecule drug candidates.

Given these differences, Saha said, there are challenging questions that require answering with regard to clinical trials for gene-based therapies. For example, he asked, what type of evidence is needed to bring a gene-based therapy into human clinical trials, and how should that evidence be collected responsibly? What should an optimal starting dose be? What are the stopping criteria? How can delivery be optimized? How can researchers engage and communicate with all of the people involved in a clinical trial, including the patients? "Ultimately, what we are hoping to hear from the folks in the room [today] are ways to improve the design of these trials," Saha said. The objectives of workshop can be found in Box 1-1.

As a way to clearly communicate the scope of this workshop during the planning process, the planning committee used the following definition of gene therapy from FDA[3]: "[t]he administration of genetic material to modify or manipulate the expression of a gene product or to alter the biological properties of living cells for therapeutic use." For the purposes of workshop planning, the committee also considered any use of gene editing (including techniques such as CRISPR/Cas9 that allow for precise changes in the nucleic acids of a person, animal, or other living organism) to be a gene-based therapy.

ORGANIZATION OF THE WORKSHOP AND PROCEEDINGS

This Proceedings of a Workshop summarizes the presentations and discussions that took place at the workshop. The opening keynote lecture by Katherine High is covered later in this chapter, and Chapter 2 explores the early stages of development of gene-based therapies, including designing research questions and collecting preclinical data. Also included in

---

BOX 1-1
Workshop Objectives

- To gain a better understanding of the design complexities and ethical issues associated with clinical trials for gene-based therapies by considering topics such as:
  - Transitioning to first-in-human trials
  - Determining the optimal starting dose
  - Optimizing therapeutic delivery
  - Communicating risks and benefits to patients and families
- To identify potential ways to improve the design of gene therapy clinical trials from the perspective of participants, product developers, regulators, and other key stakeholders

---

[3]See What Is Gene Therapy? at https://www.fda.gov/vaccines-blood-biologics/cellular-gene-therapy-products/what-gene-therapy (accessed January 12, 2020).

Chapter 2 is a discussion of challenges with transitioning to first-in-human clinical trials. Chapter 3 addresses ethical issues surrounding patient selection, enrollment, and consent for gene-based therapies and how these issues differ from those surrounding conventional clinical trials. The discussion in this section of the proceedings also touches on resources available to help patients and providers accurately understand the potential risks and benefits of participating in a gene-based clinical trial and explores communication strategies aimed at helping patients make informed decisions about participating in trials for gene-based therapies. Chapter 3 also includes a series of patient and family perspectives on these issues. Chapter 4 presents some lessons learned from the successes and challenges of accurately measuring clinical endpoints and outcomes for gene-based therapies and moving products through the translational pathway. Chapter 5 addresses the implications of the long-term follow-up and clinical management of patients who participate in gene-based clinical trials and discusses how data from a limited number of patients can be effectively used to determine if a gene-based therapy is safe and effective. Chapter 6 includes several stakeholder perspectives on possible approaches to supporting the clinical development of safe and effective gene-based therapies going forward. The final chapter also includes a summary of lessons learned and topics discussed throughout the workshop.

LESSONS FROM THE DEVELOPMENT OF A GENE THERAPY TO TREAT CHILDREN AND ADULTS WITH INHERITED VISION LOSS

There are several challenges that gene-based therapy developers face in bringing a product to market, according to Katherine High, the president and head of research and development at Spark Therapeutics. During her keynote lecture High shared examples of these challenges and spoke about her experience with obtaining FDA approval for the first gene therapy for a genetic disease, in this case a rare inherited retinal dystrophy that goes by several names, including Leber congenital amaurosis and retinitis pigmentosa (Russell et al., 2017).

In the United States, 1,000 to 2,000 individuals have this disease, which is caused by an autosomal recessive mutation in a gene called retinal pigment epithelium 65 kilodalton protein (*RPE65*), High explained. It is characterized by the early onset of retinal degeneration and nyctalopia or "night blindness." High said that many of these patients are identified during infancy by parents who notice their infant cannot visually track or follow an object or that the infant experiences involuntary eye movements (nystagmus). By the second decade of life, nearly everyone with this disorder has significant visual impairment and over time, most people with the condition will progress to blindness (Chung et al., 2019).

When the team at Spark Therapeutics first started this project, High said, there was no treatment for any inherited retinal dystrophy, but there was compelling evidence that subretinal injection of an adeno-associated virus (AAV) vector expressing the correct form of *RPE65* could restore vision in a naturally occurring dog model of the disease (Acland et al., 2001; Bennicelli et al., 2008). In 2007 the Spark team initiated dose-escalation Phase 1 trials in the eye with the worst function in 12 adult and pediatric patients (see Figure 1-1). This study showed that even the highest dose of the *RPE65*-carrying viral vector was safe, and the higher dose was then injected into the opposite (previously untreated with this viral vector) eyes of the 12 test subjects.

Using Natural History Data in Clinical Trials

In addition to the clinical trials of AAV2-*RPE65*, FDA encouraged the company to conduct a natural history study in patients with biallelic *RPE65* mutation-associated retinal dystrophy; the data from such studies can be useful in interpreting safety and efficacy data generated from a trial. High said that natural history data, if robust, can be used as a control group for a clinical trial, although in the case of retinitis pigmentosa the available natural history data were mainly from single-institution case reports and therefore were not convincing enough to be used in this way. The research team attempted to overcome this challenge by conducting a natural history study in parallel to the Phase 3 trial. The natural history study involved a retrospective chart review of patients who had a genetically confirmed diagnosis and at least two office visits. By working with seven referral centers on three continents,

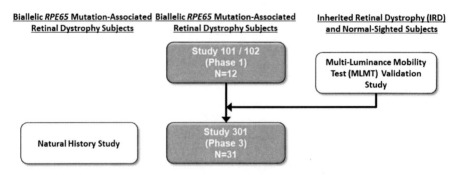

FIGURE 1-1 Clinical development of AAV2-*RPE65* (Luxturna).
SOURCES: Katherine High workshop presentation, November 13, 2019. Originally from https://www.fda.gov/media/108680/download (accessed March 30, 2020).

High and her colleagues developed a database of 70 individuals ranging in age from 1 to 43 who met the inclusion criteria, from which they were able to construct curves describing the loss of individuals' visual field and visual acuity over time (Chung et al., 2019; Holladay, 1997).

Understanding Important Characteristics of the Study Population

In studies of genetic diseases, High said, it is important that the study design call for verifying the genetic diagnosis in each individual and for being aware of any genotype or phenotype correlations that may affect safety or efficacy. For a progressively degenerative disease such as this one, it is important to stratify the Phase 3 randomization process based on disease stage and severity. For the Phase 3 trial of AAV2-RPE65, the two arms were balanced in terms of the number of subjects less than 10 years old and those 10 years of age and older (as a proxy for disease progression/severity) and also in the subjects' ability to pass the primary endpoint, the mobility test, above or below a defined level of illumination at baseline (Russell et al., 2017).

Ethical Considerations with Pediatric Subjects

Because the preclinical studies in dogs had demonstrated that the earlier the intervention, the better the eventual outcome, the research team wanted to include children in the clinical trials from the start. However, High said, if including children in an interventional trial involves more than minimal risk,[4] the trial has to offer the prospect of direct clinical benefit for every child enrolled. The Children's Hospital of Philadelphia's institutional review board (IRB) deemed that because the administration procedure involved general anesthesia, removal of some or all of the fluid inside the eye, and subretinal injection, the trial clearly involved more than minimal risk. As a result, the Phase 1/2 trial design called for starting with a dose at which the majority of affected eyes in the dog study recovered vision and then escalating from there. Federal regulatory bodies agreed.

Developing and Validating Efficacy Endpoints

Regulators at FDA asked High and her team to also conduct a validation study in normal subjects and in those with inherited retinal dystrophies in order to assess the performance characteristics of the multi-luminance

---

[4]Federal regulations define minimal risks based on the risks "ordinarily encountered in daily life or during routine physical or psychological examinations or tests" (Wendler et al., 2005, p. 827).

mobility test (MLMT) (the primary endpoint in Phase 3) that they had devised in close dialogue with FDA. (Additional details on the development of the multi-luminance mobility test are discussed by Albert Maguire in Chapter 4.) High noted that FDA's 2018 draft guidance document on human gene therapy trials for rare diseases emphasizes the importance of discussing primary efficacy endpoints with FDA because well-established, disease-specific efficacy endpoints are not available for many rare diseases.

The MLMT, a mobility test conducted at a series of light levels, served as a novel primary efficacy endpoint for inherited retinal dystrophy caused by *RPE65* mutations. In the separate validation study, which compared performance in both sighted participants and those with inherited retinal dystrophies, the investigators found that no subjects with an inherited retinal dystrophy improved over the course of 1 year without treatment and that in 28 percent of these subjects the condition worsened.

Points to Consider with Gene Therapy Trial Design

A randomized controlled crossover trial design was used for the Phase 3 clinical trial of AAV2-*RPE65*. A two-to-one randomization was used so that people would sign up knowing that they had a two-thirds chance of being part of the intervention, High noted. Using such a design would be more difficult for diseases that are fatal, she said. In those cases, alternative clinical trial designs are needed, with the exact trial design depending on if there are alternative treatments available and if the disease is currently treated by a complex medical regimen but one with decades of clinical experiences, as is the case with hemophilia.

However, by day 30 of the trial it was clear that those in the intervention group were seeing marked improvement in their ability to maneuver quickly and accurately in dim light compared with the control subjects. As the study progressed, that improvement persisted for 1 year, and members of the control group became eligible to receive the intervention as part of the crossover clinical trial design. Those in the control group that crossed over to receive the intervention experienced the same benefits as the original intervention group. Members of both groups also experienced marked improvement in their visual fields after receiving the intervention. When asked if patients receiving the lowest dose were allowed to receive a second, higher dose, High replied that large animal studies suggest that re-administration should be safe. However, she reminded the audience that studies of other gene therapies have found that animal studies are poor predictors of human immune response to the viral vector used to deliver the gene. "I think that represents a risk that would have to have, in my opinion, a strongly worded consent form to re-administer to the same eye," she said. She also noted that there is a dose-dependent risk of triggering an inflammatory response in the eye.

In closing, High said that understanding the pathophysiology and natural history of the disease played a critical role in developing the clinical endpoint because it led to measuring mobility at different levels of illumination, something that existing mobility tests did not do. High noted, too, that collecting clinical measurements repeatedly over time can yield important information, which is why the Spark clinical trial collected data at baseline, 30 days, 90 days, 180 days, and 365 days.

2

Developing First-in-Human Gene Therapy Clinical Trials

<table>
<tr><td colspan="2" align="center">Important Points Highlighted by Individual Speakers</td></tr>
<tr><td>•</td><td>Understanding the nuances of genotype and phenotype associations can help with designing an efficient clinical trial, specifically in the case of pediatric studies that may require different outcome measures and study designs. Genetic diagnoses are also important to know upfront because they may affect the safety and efficacy of an experimental gene therapy. (Finkel, Kaufmann)</td></tr>
<tr><td>•</td><td>For certain diseases that are in both pediatric and adult populations, it may make sense to carry out early clinical trials in the pediatric population, especially if it is known that early treatment improves overall outcomes. (Finkel)</td></tr>
<tr><td>•</td><td>Robust natural history datasets with frequent visits to the research team; standardized measures; high-quality, patient-level data; and complete follow-up are needed to develop treatments for patients with rare diseases who could benefit from gene therapy. (Kaufmann)</td></tr>
<tr><td>•</td><td>During the clinical development process, sponsors should engage with patient advocacy groups because they can provide an important perspective on regulatory, recruitment, and research and trial design issues. (Kaufmann)</td></tr>
</table>

- Decisions about risk versus benefit are ultimately ethical judgments made by ethics committees and institutional review boards (IRBs), but many IRBs do not spend enough time carefully vetting preclinical evidence and may not be well equipped in terms of technical expertise. (Kimmelman)

The challenges that arise in the design of early-stage clinical trials for gene-based therapies was the topic of the workshop's first session, which was moderated by Cindy Dunbar, a senior investigator at the National Heart, Lung, and Blood Institute (NHLBI). Richard Finkel, the neurology division chief in the Department of Pediatrics at Nemours Children's Health System, spoke about natural history studies for Duchenne muscular dystrophy (DMD) and spinal muscular atrophy. Petra Kaufmann, the vice president for translational medicine at AveXis, reviewed the development of gene therapy for spinal muscular atrophy. Jonathan Kimmelman, the director of the biomedical ethics unit at McGill University, provided an overview of the ethical dimensions and recurrent challenges associated with early-phase research and first-in-human trials.

USING NATURAL HISTORY STUDIES IN CLINICAL DEVELOPMENT

When developing a clinical trial in a pediatric population, sponsors should carefully consider the study population and whether it includes newborns, infants, children, or adolescents, Finkel said. Key differences exist among these subgroups, such as differences in the volume of blood and cerebral spinal fluid in the body, which affect drug delivery and target engagement, as well as weight differences, which can affect dosing. Drug metabolism and excretion can differ as a child ages, which can affect drug exposure and a drug's safety profile, and off-target effects may differ in children of different ages. A disease can also present differently in pediatric and adult populations, Finkel noted, so different outcome measures and study designs would be required for these two populations.

If a disease is present in both the adult and pediatric population, it is typical that clinical trials will take place first in the adult population, Finkel said, but he questioned whether this precaution is necessary. In certain situations, he said, there are persuasive arguments to start in children, especially if it is known that early treatment makes a difference, but an ethical challenge arises if a disease first appears in infants and the aim is to generate the most robust response to a drug.

DMD offers an example of why it is important to understand the natural history of a disease when thinking about gene therapy clinical trial designs, Finkel said. DMD is an X chromosome–linked genetic disorder that affects 1 in 3,500 boys, with an onset between ages 2 and 4 years old.[1] Historically, boys with this disorder often lost their ability to walk by age 10, and almost none of those with the disorder were able to walk past age 13. Today, however, steroids can extend ambulation by about 3 years, Finkel said. Furthermore, the specific mutation that an individual carries plays a major role in functional outcomes, with some patients not losing ambulation until 20 years of age (Wang et al., 2018). It is critically important to understand the genotype–phenotype relationship when clinical trials are being designed, Finkel said.

As a second example, Finkel discussed spinal muscular atrophy (SMA), in which two genes—*SMN1* and *SMN2*—play a role. Children missing a functional copy of *SMN1* depend on the small amount of protein produced by *SMN2*, which prevents fetal lethality but is insufficient to prevent the progressive disorder from occurring. Because two genes are involved, there are two possible treatment strategies. One approach, taken by Biogen with its antisense oligonucleotide drug Spinraza®, modifies the *SMN2* gene so that it produces more functional protein, Finkel said. Spinraza® was the first drug approved by FDA to treat SMA, and is delivered via intrathecal injection with four loading doses. Risdiplam is another SMA therapy that modifies the *SMN2* gene in a similar way to Spinraza®, but the small molecule is orally active. Risdiplam is currently under clinical investigation by Roche, PTC Therapeutics, and the Spinal Muscular Atrophy Foundation.

The second approach, which AveXis took in developing the gene replacement therapy Zolgensma®, is a more traditional gene therapy approach where a single intravenous dose delivers a corrected copy of the *SMN1* gene in order to replace the non-functional or missing copy of the gene, Finkel said. Zolgensma® received FDA approval in 2019 for use in children under 2 years of age.[2] Because Spinraza® was available as an approved product, it was possible to conduct a randomized controlled trial for Zolgensma® with Spinraza® as the comparison control, Finkel said.

Transitioning to the topic of early-stage research and how those findings can help prepare for clinical trials, Finkel touched on the importance of animal models. Shortly after the *SMN* genes were identified by Judith

---

[1] For a more thorough review of genetic changes in Duchenne muscular dystrophy and the implications for therapy, see Gao and McNally (2015).

[2] See FDA News Release at https://www.fda.gov/news-events/press-announcements/fda-approves-innovative-gene-therapy-treat-pediatric-patients-spinal-muscular-atrophy-rare-disease (accessed January 26, 2020).

Melki and colleagues in 1995, researchers recognized the need for animal models to study the disease, he said. Arthur Burghes and his colleagues generated a knockout mouse model containing a human *SMN2* transgene that recapitulates the severe type 1 form of SMA and predicts response to drugs (Monani et al., 2000). In the years that followed, Finkel said, additional models of SMA were developed and characterized in zebrafish (McWhorter et al., 2003), flies (Chan et al., 2003), and, more recently, pigs (Duque et al., 2015).

On the clinical side, researchers found that disease severity was reduced in children who have additional copies of the *SMN2* gene (Feldkötter et al., 2002). Finkel and his colleagues went on to show that infants with the most severe form of the disease (Type 1, or Werdnig-Hoffmann disease) who had two copies of *SMN2* exhibited greater morbidity and mortality than infants who carried three copies of the *SMN2* gene (Finkel et al., 2014). Furthermore, Finkel and his collaborators developed outcome measures that assessed motor function, strength, and weakness (Finkel et al., 2014) as well as electrophysiological markers (Swoboda et al., 2005) and a neuro-filament marker (Darras et al., 2019) in order to predict the disease course in untreated and treated patients.

Natural history studies of SMA patients were valuable because they showed that age is an important variable with regard to the change in motor function, Finkel said, and there was significant functional variability among the ambulant patient population (Mercuri et al., 2016). There is a need to understand the characteristics of the patient population and to notice that certain subgroups are more amenable to change without drugs, he said. When one drug candidate, valproic acid, was tested in young children, the improvement seen in some of the children was apparently not a result of the drug but instead was due to variations in the natural history of the disease. The standard of care (which can involve non-invasive ventilation support, nutritional support, physical therapy, and other interventions) produced a marked improvement in survival from the 1980s into the 1990s without any drug therapy, Finkel said, and is another factor to consider when designing a clinical trial (De Sanctis et al., 2016; Oskoui et al., 2007).

Currently, Finkel said, a Phase 3 open-label trial using a historical control is under way with Zolgensma®. Zolgensma® (also known as AVXS-101) is being tested in symptomatic infants with SMA type 1, the severe form of the disease. Data so far have shown that this therapy produces a marked improvement in event-free survival, Finkel said, with those children who are treated as soon as symptoms appear responding best to the gene replacement. Treatment shortly after birth in the pre-symptomatic period appears to generate the most robust response not only with Zolgensma®, but also in the case of Spinraza® and Risdiplam.

In the gene therapy development process, it is helpful to talk to FDA early and often, Finkel said, adding that a paper written by a group of FDA staff (Xu et al., 2017) was helpful in summarizing important lessons about the development of gene therapies, specifically from the perspective of developing Spinraza®. In summary, Finkel said that pediatric studies have particular challenges and regulatory requirements and that understanding the nuances of genotype and phenotype associations can help in the design of an efficient clinical trial. It is necessary to provide standard of care to minimize patient variation, he said, but this adds a second treatment variable to any clinical trial.

DEVELOPMENT OF GENE THERAPY FOR SPINAL MUSCULAR ATROPHY

Continuing on the topic of SMA, Kaufmann said that this disorder affects approximately 1 in 10,000 live births worldwide and that around 1 in 54 people carry the genetic defect responsible for causing this disease (Mendell et al., 2017). The *SMN2* modifying gene plays a role in determining the phenotypic severity of the disease, with the most severe form affecting infants and with milder forms that may even present as late as adulthood. Approximately 60 percent of individuals with SMA have type 1 disease, the most severe form, and these individuals show symptoms before age 6 months and are never are able to sit up, and most never see their second birthday. In type 2 disease, which affects approximately 30 percent of patients and first appears between ages 6 and 18 months, individuals can sit, but are never able to walk, and more than 30 percent of these individuals will die by the time they are 25. In type 3 disease, accounting for about 10 percent of patients, individuals can walk but may lose that ability over time (Lorson et al., 2010; Verhaart et al., 2017). Type 1 disease, because of its severity and lethality, was the strongest candidate for the first gene therapy trial, Kaufmann said.

There are different types of natural history data available on SMA patients, Kaufmann said. She and her colleagues at AveXis used patient registries and associated medical charts to get an initial understanding of the course of the disease, she said, noting that these data sources do have significant limitations, particularly missing data or limited time course data. To get a fuller picture of the natural history of type 1 disease, Kaufmann collaborated with Finkel and his colleagues and a group at Columbia University on a cross-sectional and prospective natural history study (Finkel et al., 2014).

Researchers were grateful for the patients and families who participated in this study because they made a significant time commitment to the study and recognized that there might not be direct benefit for their families,

Kaufmann said. She added that it would have been better to have a fully prospective study with regular, more frequent visits, but that would have placed an even greater burden on patients and their families. Later, the National Institutes of Health did fund a more complete, prospective natural history study of type 1 SMA by the Network for Excellence in Neuroscience Clinical Trials (NeuroNEXT),[3] which confirmed what she and her colleagues had found. The NeuroNEXT natural history study also provided more data on changes in motor function and electrophysiological measures that were fit for use in clinical trials (Kolb et al., 2017).

One of the important breakthroughs that enabled gene therapy trials for diseases that affect the central nervous system, Kaufmann said, was the discovery that AAV vectors can cross the blood–brain barrier and robustly express transported genes in cells throughout the brain and spinal cord (Foust et al., 2009). This vector was used to design a construct that would enable immediate and sustained expression of the *SMN1* protein and produce a rapid onset and durable therapeutic effect, the latter of which was possible because the vector targets non-dividing neurons. The vector was also designed not to integrate into the human genome (Naso et al., 2017; Thomas et al., 2003).

In the Phase 1 clinical trial, three patients were given what was thought to be the minimally effective dose based on animal studies, and another 12 patients were given the proposed therapeutic dose (Mendell et al., 2017). There was an initial 2-year safety follow-up period, and the patients will be followed for another 15 years. "In a new field it is critical that we have a good understanding of what happens to the patients in the long term," Kaufmann said. The patients who received the gene therapy construct had improved survival, motor function, and motor milestone achievements, she said, and the patients treated with the proposed therapeutic dose had early and rapid motor function improvements.

At 24 months following the gene therapy administration, all patients were alive and did not need permanent ventilation, and 11 of 12 patients in the therapeutic dose group could sit without assistance for longer than 5 seconds. Furthermore, two patients in that cohort were able to stand and walk independently, and so far, patients who received the therapeutic dose continue to achieve and maintain motor function milestones, Kaufmann said. As Finkel had noted, Zolgensma® was approved by FDA in May 2019 for the treatment of pediatric patients under age 2 years who have mutations in the *SMN1* gene. Subsequent studies have shown that it is best to treat patients at a very young age, even before they display symptoms.

---

[3] For more information on NeuroNEXT, see https://neuronext.org (accessed January 26, 2020).

In conclusion, Kaufmann said, robust natural history data with frequent visits are important for developing treatments for patients with rare disease who could benefit from gene therapy. Directly engaging with patient groups that can help with recruitment and represent the patient perspective in regulatory and drug development contexts was incredibly important, she added. Finally, she reiterated how important the altruistic participation of patients and families in natural history studies is for the development of efficient gene therapy clinical trials.

ETHICAL DIMENSIONS OF FIRST-IN-HUMAN GENE TRANSFER TRIALS

Kimmelman provided a high-level overview of research ethics and discussed those concepts within the context of gene therapy clinical trials. Research that is conducted in humans is ethically challenging because human beings can feel pain, suffer, and have their own interests, Kimmelman said. One purpose of research on humans is to generate information that will be useful for other people in the future. As a result, an important aspect of research ethics involves ensuring that trial-generated information does not get adulterated, either during the study or when health care systems take up that information. Another important aspect of research ethics focuses on the highly trained and specialized individuals who conduct research on human beings, Kimmelman said. This highly trained workforce should be concentrating on the most productive lines of research in order to generate highly reliable information about the safety and efficacy of a particular treatment. Doing so may help to ensure that health care dollars are not wasted on expensive and ineffective therapies, he said.

All potential drugs, including gene therapies, need to undergo an arduous vetting process of clinical development and be proven safe and effective, Kimmelman said. The first stage in the development process is considered a learning phase in which researchers try to determine how best to use the therapy. For example, developing a cell-based therapy for amyotrophic lateral sclerosis requires knowing the appropriate dose of cells to deliver, the type of immunosuppression regimen required, and the timing of the drug administration that achieves optimal benefit.

The next task, Kimmelman said, is to use this information to design and conduct rigorous clinical evaluations, typically randomized controlled trials. Deciding when to initiate early-phase clinical trials requires a basic understanding of the potential risks and benefits of the proposed treatment, and that in turn involves demonstrating potential efficacy and safety in high-quality preclinical studies. In the case of gene and cell therapies, FDA pays closer attention to the quality and design of preclinical studies (e.g., blinding and the selection of appropriate controls) than it does for small molecule drugs, Kimmelman said. Ultimately though, broader decisions about risk versus benefit are ethical judgments made by IRBs and ethics committees, he said, and FDA is clear about delegating those types of ethical judgments. One problem with this approach, he said, is that some IRBs may not be well equipped to carefully vet all of the preclinical evidence and to make judgments about the prospect of direct and societal benefits.

Another recurrent challenge in the conduct of early-phase research is deciding whether to consider exposure to the new intervention to be therapeutic. There are two main reasons why it does not make sense to call access to interventions and early-phase studies therapeutic, Kimmelman said. The first is that during the early stages of clinical research it is not yet clear if an intervention will be effective because the goal during this phase is to identify the materials, practices, and beliefs needed to combine with an intervention to elicit its activity. Claims of therapeutic benefit in first-in-human clinical trials should be met with skepticism, Kimmelman said. A second reason it does not make sense to call early-phase clinical studies therapeutic, he said, is that there is not strong evidence to suggest that participation in an early-phase clinical trial will provide any therapeutic benefit, given that most early-phase research studies fail to find evidence of efficacy and safety. In his own research, Kimmelman said, he has observed that the fraction of patients who enter a Phase 1 clinical trial and receive a drug at a dose that will ultimately receive FDA approval for their indication is about 1 in 70, while 10 to 15 percent of participants in a Phase 1 trial will experience a grade 3 or grade 4 adverse event (unpublished finding).

Looking beyond an assessment of safety, Kimmelman said that a major challenge of early research studies is to define the lowest effective dose and the optimal timing of delivery, particularly for interventions that are expected to be expensive, such as gene-based therapies. Another challenge is to avoid conducting an uninformative trial—that is, one that does not provide results that are of value to patients, researchers, clinicians, or policy makers (Zarin et al., 2019). Whether a trial is considered to be informative is based on its relevance, design, feasibility, integrity of analysis, and reporting (Zarin et al., 2019). In particular, reporting the results of early-phase research is critically important so that subsequent researchers or health care systems can use the data in patient decision making (Fung et al., 2017). "It is critical that we recognize that if patients have participated in clinical research, we honor their sacrifice and contribution by making sure that we are promptly and completely reporting the results of their participation," Kimmelman said.

DISCUSSION

Following the three presentations in this session, there was a panel discussion moderated by Dunbar, and workshop participants had an opportunity to ask questions of the speakers. Topics during the panel discussion included early-phase trials for pediatric patients, patient stratification, and ways to improve clinical trial readiness.

Issues with Conducting Early-Phase Trials in Pediatric Patients

There is an inherent conflict between a first-in-human trial not being considered therapeutic and the requirement to offer a pediatric population a chance of therapeutic benefit, Dunbar said. How can that be dealt with, she asked the speakers, especially with regard to consent forms? There are exceptions to the general rule against designing Phase 1 studies for therapeutic outcomes, Kimmelman said, especially when there is exceptionally detailed mechanistic data. Another potential exception would be when similar interventions have already been tried in other genetic diseases using the same (or very similar) vectors, and a safety profile is established.

When there is no treatment for a disease and there is the prospect of a gene therapy, parents will still often sign their children up for a trial because they are desperate for any improvement, Finkel said. "The real obligation, I think, is on the physician serving as the investigator to frame the discussion carefully and look at the risk and benefit," he said, adding that his institution has a policy where a patient advocate is present in his discussions with parents to make sure that he and other investigators are presenting information in an unbiased manner and that parents are truly understanding the potential benefits and risks. Kaufmann agreed that it is critical to be transparent with parents and to have good information available for them. "I think the more we partner with patients, the more we have strong patient groups who can provide that kind of information to parents and patients, the better off we are," she said.

Data Collection and Patient Stratification

Speakers were asked whether they believed clinical trial data collection was robust enough to be able to understand which patients are most likely to benefit (or not benefit) from the therapy. The more information that researchers can collect, Kaufmann said, the better chance they have of being able to stratify patients in the future. The therapies being discussed in this session apply to a very small group of the broader population, Finkel said, and it is not clear how generalizable the results are, even when the therapy is highly effective in the study population. Once a drug is commercially available, real-world data from registries can be collected, he added, which can be very valuable for understanding patient stratification.

Tools and Approaches Useful for Clinical Trial Readiness

Speakers were asked by a workshop participant if they could identify tools or models that they have found useful in their work, specifically for determining the minimal effective dose of a gene therapy. High answered that large animal models are very useful in predicting therapeutic doses, efficacy, and safety. Kaufmann agreed, adding that forming partnerships with patient groups and potential investigators early, while preclinical work is ongoing, is helpful for trial readiness. Finkel said that his group has been finding it useful to develop informative biomarkers for early readouts regarding safety and efficacy.

The topic of continuous monitoring devices was brought up by a workshop participant, who asked the speakers if they were considering those types of approaches as a way to collect frequent data from patients. This is an area that needs to be explored, Kaufmann said, especially for use with patients who may need to travel for treatment and assessment. Such technology would also provide data from patients in their natural environment, as opposed to the clinical environment. The challenge, she said, is dealing with the flood of data that such devices would generate. Patient privacy might also be an issue with such devices. Another challenge, High said, will be to correlate the data from wearable devices with more standard measures.

Exploring Future Opportunities and Challenges

A workshop participant asked if there were procedural and ethical differences between gene-based therapies and cell-based therapies. High answered that viral vectors used to deliver gene therapies, such as AAV, are similar to other specialty pharmaceuticals in that they are manufactured and shipped to a pharmacy, whereas cell therapies require a far more complicated infrastructure that resembles that used for bone marrow transplants. There are concerns, she said, that if a cell-based therapy for a disease such as sickle cell disease works, creating the infrastructure to treat as many as 100,000 people could be difficult.

Panelists were asked if they see gene therapies being used in the future for more common, chronic diseases such as osteoarthritis. It will take a great deal of experience and safety data from rare disease indications before the field will start thinking about more common chronic diseases, Kaufmann said. There will also be the problem of scalability that will require innovation in manufacturing processes to address. Dunbar noted, however, that gene therapy is already being used in the cancer field.

Speakers were asked if it might be possible to use the results from one trial in a rare disease to shorten the development time for a similar disease, say all retinal diseases, rather than starting from zero for each disease. High responded that timelines for clinical development have shortened over the 30 years that gene therapy clinical trials have been run, and she said that FDA's draft guidance documents issued in 2018[4] should help further shorten timelines.

---

[4]See Cellular and Gene Therapy Guidances at https://www.fda.gov/vaccines-blood-biologics/ biologics-guidances/cellular-gene-therapy-guidances (accessed January 26, 2020).

3

Understanding the Complexities of Patient Selection, Enrollment, and the Consent Process

Important Points Highlighted by Individual Speakers

- Gene therapy approaches to sickle cell disease allow patients to serve as their own donors, eliminating the need for immuno-suppression and the risk of graft-versus-host disease. However, there is a need for better long-term follow-up data to compare success rates of gene therapy versus cell-based therapies such as bone marrow transplants in order to know which approach has better outcomes. (Fitzhugh, Tisdale)
- Patients should be considered partners in the clinical develop-ment process, and returning the results of a clinical trial back to the participants is an important area of the therapeutic development process that needs to be improved. (Tisdale)
- Newborn screening for severe combined immunodeficiency is critical because it provides an unbiased population-level ability to make an early diagnosis, which in turn promotes fair access to treatments, including clinical trials. (Puck)
- There is some concern that children who undergo gene therapy for Duchenne muscular dystrophy might require retreatment when they are older as muscle cells turn over. Determining when to deliver subsequent doses of gene therapy is impor-tant, given that waiting until symptoms appear might result in irreparable damage. (Furlong)

- From the family perspective on gene therapy clinical trials, safety is an important concern, but because some diseases have no approved treatments, families may be willing to take on substantial risks. The paradigm of starting clinical trials in adults or only in symptomatic patients to prove safety should change, especially given that time is of the essence for pediatric patients. (Bartek)
- The creation of a common manufacturing facility that would have the capacity to provide sufficient material for small Phase 1 gene therapy clinical trials by academic investigators would be beneficial for the field because it would not require a significant financial investment from pharmaceutical companies. (Bartek)
- The National Center for Advancing Translational Sciences and the Food and Drug Administration should consider collaborating on the development of a standardized clinical trial design that would apply to rare diseases. (Bartek)
- A sensitive issue for many families considering a gene therapy clinical trial is that there are no protocols for treating affected siblings. (Contreras)
- Regulatory agencies should consider developing innovative protocols that minimize placebo arms and allow the use of natural history studies, master protocols that may combine different therapeutic approaches, and more involvement of patients and families in protocol design. (Contreras)
- Consent forms for gene-based therapy clinical trials are too complicated to be understood in a single reading, and researchers should build in extra time to answer questions. Patients may need to process the information on their own and with their families and support networks. (Fitzhugh, Puck, Samuels)

The workshop's second session explored the ethical issues surrounding patient selection, enrollment, and consent for gene-based therapies and how those differ from conventional clinical trials. This session also identified resources that can help patients and providers accurately understand the potential risks and benefits of participating in a gene-based clinical trial and explored communication strategies aimed at helping patients make informed decisions about participating in trials for gene-based therapies. The discussion was moderated by Mildred Cho, a research professor of pediatrics and the associate director of the Center for Biomedical Ethics at Stanford University. Courtney Fitzhugh, a Lasker clinical research scholar in the Laboratory of Early Sickle Mortality Prevention at NHLBI, discussed the complexities of patient selection, enrollment, and consent in the context of hematopoietic stem cell transplantation to treat sickle cell disease, while John Tisdale, a senior investigator and the director of the Cellular and Molecular Therapeutics Laboratory at NHLBI, did the same for gene therapies for sickle cell disease. Jennifer Puck, a professor in the pediatrics department at the University of California, San Francisco, addressed these issues in the context of gene therapy for severe combined immunodeficiency (SCID) in the Navajo population. Pat Furlong, the founding president and the chief executive officer of Parent Project Muscular Dystrophy, provided a patient perspective on informed consent, enrollment, and other ethical issues surrounding gene therapy clinical trials. Following these four presentations, there were an additional three speakers who provided patient and family perspectives: Ronald Bartek, a co-founder and the president of the Friedreich's Ataxia Research Alliance; María José Contreras, a mother of two sons with DMD; and Tesha Samuels, who participated in a gene-based sickle cell disease clinical trial run by Tisdale in 2018. An open discussion with the panelists followed these presentations.

THE COMPLEXITIES OF PATIENT SELECTION, ENROLLMENT, AND CONSENT IN THE CONTEXT OF HEMATOPOIETIC STEM CELL TRANSPLANTATION TO TREAT SICKLE CELL DISEASE

Sickle cell disease, Fitzhugh explained, is caused by a point mutation that causes the hemoglobin protein to polymerize upon deoxygenation, which in turn triggers the transformation of red blood cells from flexible, biconcave disks to rigid, sickle-shaped cells that can block capillaries and small veins. Sickling episodes can occur at any time, and they cause debilitating pain, strokes, liver disease, retinopathy that can lead to blindness, painful leg ulcers, avascular necrosis, and organ damage (Thein and Howard, 2018). Patients with sickle cell disease tend to need hip replacements at a young age, are more prone to develop infections, and often suffer from kidney failure requiring dialysis. Fitzhugh said that the survival rate of children with sickle cell disease has improved substantially since the late 1970s, largely thanks to newborn screening, penicillin prophylaxis, and pneumococcal vaccination. However, the median age at death for adults with sickle cell disease (age 46 in a recent cohort) has changed little over the past 40 years (Fitzhugh et al., 2015; Hassell, 2010).

For individuals with sickle cell disease, hematopoietic stem cell transplantation offers a curative option. The most common type of transplant, Fitzhugh said, uses a sibling who is a complete tissue match as a donor to completely replace the patient's bone marrow with that of the donor. One study of 1,000 patients with sickle cell disease who underwent myeloablative chemotherapy pretreatment and matched sibling transplants found that in adults the 5-year overall survival rate was 92.9 percent and event-free survival was 91.4 percent, while for patients younger than age 16 the corresponding rates were 95 percent and 93 percent (Gluckman et al., 2017). However, the cumulative incidence of grades II–IV acute graft-versus-host disease (GVHD) was 14.8 percent and the rate of chronic GVHD was 14.3 percent—an unacceptably high incidence of a condition that can cause hardening of the skin, lung scarring, and death. In treating sickle cell disease, the goal is to avoid GVHD because it can potentially be worse for the patients, Fitzhugh said. In addition, many adults who already have organ damage cannot tolerate the myeloablative process.

To overcome this problem, Fitzhugh worked with Tisdale to develop a regimen that uses alemtuzumab, a medication for treating chronic lymphocytic leukemia, to suppress the immune system and deplete it of lymphocytes for 1 month, combined with low-dose total body irradiation to make space in the bone marrow and provide additional immunosuppression. The regimen also includes the drug sirolimus, a compound with immunosuppressive, antitumor, and antiviral properties, in an attempt to mitigate the risk of GVHD. A key difference between this regimen and the standard one with myeloablative chemotherapy is that this one does not completely replace the patient's bone marrow with that of the donor, and, indeed, Fitzhugh said, it is not necessary to replace all of the bone marrow to cure sickle cell disease. The key, she said, is to have at least 20 percent of the red blood cells coming from the donor. "That is because of the vast differences in half-lives between a normal red cell, which lasts about 3 months, and a sickled red cell, that survives for 5 to 20 days," said Fitzhugh.

In a study examining the new regimen, none of the 55 patients who received the transplanted hematopoietic stem cells experienced GVHD, though one patient became dependent on blood transfusions for 1.5 years following the transplant, Fitzhugh said (unpublished results). In addition, seven patients rejected the graft (due to graft failure), and six of those individuals had their sickle cell disease return, with the seventh patient dying from an intracranial hemorrhage caused by her sickle cell disease. The overall survival rate was 93 percent, and event-free survival was 87 percent. Unlike the situation with the myeloablative regimen, where most patients are expected to not be able to have children on their own, 8 of the patients using this milder regimen with lower doses of irradiation have had 13 healthy babies post-transplant.

The major problem with this approach is that only about 15 percent of individuals with sickle cell disease will have a sibling who is a complete tissue match. Fitzhugh and her colleagues therefore offer haploidentical transplantation that allows parents, children, and half-matched siblings to serve as donors. The downside with haploidentical transplantation is that there is a higher risk of graft rejection and GVHD. One study of this approach found that in a cohort of 12 individuals who received two doses of cyclophosphamide post-transplant, only 6 remained free of sickle cell disease because of a relatively high rate of graft rejection (Fitzhugh et al., 2017b). However, more recent results in the haploidentical setting are much more encouraging.

Although Fitzhugh did not discuss gene therapy approaches to treat sickle cell disease—a topic that was covered by Tisdale, the following speaker—Fitzhugh did describe what she and her colleagues tell patients about gene therapy. To start, she tells them, patients can serve as their own donors, which means that it should be available to all patients. There is no need for immunosuppression and no risk of GVHD when the patient is the donor. Myeloablative conditioning is still necessary, and the short- and long-term success of gene therapies is not yet known. In addition, patients with significant organ damage are currently excluded from receiving gene therapy due to the need for high dose chemotherapy. After receiving this information, as well as being briefed on the pros and cons of donor bone marrow transplantation and being assessed for the severity of their disease, patients can decide whether to move forward with a transplant, and if so, what option to choose, Fitzhugh said. "We have to ensure that in each individual patient, the potential benefits outweigh the risks," she said. A common reason that patients choose gene therapy is to not inconvenience family members or put them at risk from donating bone marrow, she added.

More recent protocols at NHLBI do not include children, given that 98 percent of children with sickle cell disease will survive to age 18, making it hard to justify any procedure with a significant risk of mortality associated with it. It is difficult to explain this to patients and advise them to wait because their disease is not severe enough at that time, Fitzhugh said. In her experience, she said, even after the risks associated with transplantation have been explained to them, some patients are surprised when they reject the graft.

As a result of those experiences, Fitzhugh said, she and her colleagues worked with an ethics team to study the process of decision making by sickle cell disease patients who decide to participate in high-risk clinical research. The ethics team conducted interviews with 26 patients to evaluate motivations, the decision-making process, the patients' understanding of research, and retrospective reflections. Two-thirds of the patients were capable of clearly describing the purpose of research, and all patients were aware that transplant and gene therapy studies carry side effects and risks, including death, cancer, and GVHD. Of the 26 patients surveyed, 22 acknowledged that the treatment might not work, and the main concerns of the patients included worries that they would have an unsuccessful response and might die, that they might experience pain, and that they might suffer from long-term side effects.

Most of the patients described performing a personal risk–benefit calculation when deciding about participation, and all patients who decided to enroll cited the intolerability of their sickle cell disease or the hope for a better future without the disease. Those who declined enrollment felt that their current status was not bad enough to justify the risks of the trial, and half of the patients who did enroll cited altruistic motivations, although none reported altruism as their primary motive for participating in the clinical trial. When asked what role family, faith, and other patients played in their decision making, most patients reported that family provided moral support and reassurance. Eleven of the patients had spoken to patients who had positive outcomes, five had spoken with patients who had negative outcomes, and seven of the patients had not spoken to other patients.

THE COMPLEXITIES OF PATIENT SELECTION, ENROLLMENT, AND CONSENT IN THE CONTEXT OF GENE THERAPIES TO TREAT SICKLE CELL DISEASE

Continuing on the theme of sickle cell disease, Tisdale said that both allogeneic bone marrow transplantation and autologous gene therapy work by either replacing or repairing bone marrow stem cells so that the body produces hemoglobin that will not polymerize and cause sickling (see Figure 3-1). As Fitzhugh mentioned, it was recently found that only 20 percent of white blood cells need to come from either repaired or replaced bone marrow in order for the disease to be reversed (Fitzhugh et al., 2017a).

Tisdale described one challenging issue related to the fact that the vector his team uses to deliver the correcting gene to bone marrow cells is derived from HIV. Sickle cell disease has a higher incidence in individuals of African American descent, and when some patients with the disease learn that the vector is based on the virus that causes AIDS, he said, they may think back to the Tuskegee experiment[1] and become reluctant to participate in the trial. "The bottom line is that it takes a lot of education in the patient population and long-term follow-up of patients in a setting where they are getting care from physicians that they trust," he said.

After conducting a series of mouse and large animal studies to determine the potentially therapeutic dose of the vector–gene construct to admin-

---

[1]The Tuskegee experiment refers to a clinical study (Tuskegee Study of Untreated Syphilis in the Negro Male) conducted between 1932 and 1972 by the U.S. Public Health Service, which violated many bioethical research standards. The aim of the study was to understand the natural history of untreated syphilis; however, the African American men involved in the study did not receive complete and clear information about the study and its associated risks. Researchers also did not give study participants penicillin (a known cure for syphilis).

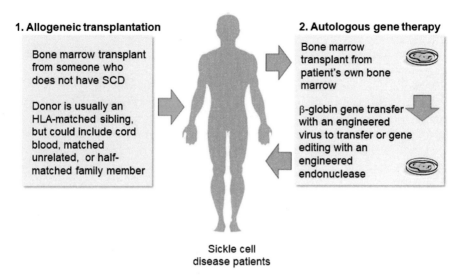

1. Allogeneic transplantation

Bone marrow transplant from someone who does not have SCD

Donor is usually an HLA-matched sibling, but could include cord blood, matched unrelated, or half-matched family member

2. Autologous gene therapy

Bone marrow transplant from patient's own bone marrow

β-globin gene transfer with an engineered virus to transfer or gene editing with an engineered endonuclease

Sickle cell
disease patients

FIGURE 3-1 Bone marrow stem cell strategies for sickle cell disease.
NOTE: HLA = human leukocyte antigen; SCD = sickle cell disease.
SOURCE: John Tisdale workshop presentation, November 13, 2019.

ister to humans, Tisdale and his colleagues designed a clinical trial to first study the construct's safety profile, with efficacy as a secondary endpoint. As the trial proceeded, he and his colleagues made several adjustments to the stem cell source and manufacturing method, which resulted in more patients experiencing improvements.

Addressing how to include pre-symptomatic individuals in clinical trials for gene therapy, Tisdale said that the field has not yet reached a place where it can consider relaxing the stringent inclusion criteria that much. "We need to know it is working, and we need to quantitate the benefit in patients for whom the risk–benefit ratio favors the intervention," he explained. "Once we have de-risked the procedure itself, or have the success rate known, then we can begin to apply that in pre-symptomatic patients."

Getting the results of the trial back to the patients who participated in it is one part of the clinical trials process that needs improving, Tisdale said. His team now makes a point of going to patient advocacy meetings and holding meetings in their clinic to update patients on the results of ongoing clinical trials. "I think it is helpful to engage the patient population as real team members in this effort," he said.

Regarding what to do if the initial application of gene therapy does not work, Tisdale said that for individuals who are in good shape, one possibility would be to follow-up with a matched sibling transplant after gene therapy fails. It would be beneficial to see long-term follow-up data comparing the success of gene therapy with the success of cell-based therapy to know if one approach is better than the other, he said.

Another approach to treating sickle cell disease involves the use of new gene-editing technologies, such as those involving CRISPR/Cas9. One gene-editing method aims to boost levels of fetal hemoglobin in individuals with sickle cell disease. In the months following birth, babies stop making fetal hemoglobin and begin to produce adult hemoglobin. Certain individuals carry genetic mutations that lead to the persistent production of fetal hemo-globin, said Tisdale, and in someone with sickle cell disease these mutations are protective and result in a very mild form of the disease because fetal hemoglobin does not polymerize and cause sickling (NIH Director's Blog, 2019). Although it is more difficult than turning the production of fetal hemoglobin back on, another gene-editing approach aims to correct the mutation that causes sickle cell disease (see Figure 3-2), Tisdale said, and his group has shown that it can correct approximately 30 percent of the hemo-globin genes and deactivate another 60 percent of the faulty hemoglobin genes, leaving only 10 percent of the faulty hemoglobin. "The majority of the hemoglobin in these red cells are now the correctly spelled beta globin protein," he said, "and this is far in excess of the 20 percent we need to fix this disease."

To explore how gene editing would be received by stakeholders, one group of investigators convened 15 focus groups in seven U.S. cities to

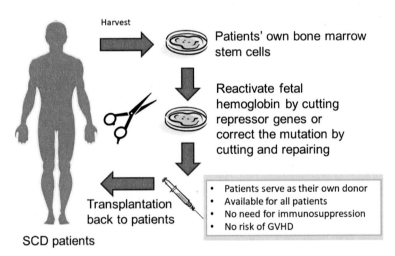

FIGURE 3-2 Autologous bone marrow stem cell–targeted gene editing to treat sickle cell disease.
NOTE: GVHD = graft-versus-host disease; SCD = sickle cell disease.
SOURCE: John Tisdale workshop presentation, November 13, 2019.

explore attitudes and beliefs toward gene editing within the sickle cell disease community (Hollister et al., 2019; Persaud et al., 2019). Focus groups were shown a short educational video on somatic genome editing and its potential use for sickle cell disease and then given a survey related to genome editing and participation in future clinical trials. The survey was followed up by open discussion periods with the researchers. According to these studies, the factors that motivated people to participate in a gene-editing trial included hope in technology, altruism, the shortcomings of current treatment, and increased awareness of the importance of clinical trials. Deterrents included uncertainty about the consequences of gene editing, the permanence of the change to the genome, trial burden, patients' mistrust of the medical community, reproductive risk, cost, and a lack of access. Mediating factors included religiosity and the capacity to manage disease and life. Patients reported that they wanted specific details about the trial, the expected interpatient variability, optimal timing, and the track record of the treatment. On a final note, Tisdale stressed that he had been talking about somatic cell–based gene therapy and gene editing, not working with germ-line cells, and that the National Institutes of Health (NIH) has been clear that none of this work will use human embryos.

THE COMPLEXITIES OF PATIENT SELECTION, ENROLLMENT, AND CONSENT IN THE CONTEXT OF GENE THERAPY FOR SEVERE COMBINED IMMUNODEFICIENCY

SCID, a condition in which the body cannot fight infections because it cannot mount an immune response, can result from defects in many genes, Puck told the workshop audience. Babies born with this disease start to lose weight from age 2 to 4 months, and they will not survive unless given a working immune system. This was first accomplished in 1968, when an infant boy with SCID received the first successful bone marrow transplant, using his sister as the donor. This boy is now a 52-year-old man who is healthy and was able to father a child, said Puck.

Because individuals with SCID do not have a working immune system, donors can be parents, matched unrelated donors, or cord blood, Puck said. One form of SCID, characterized by adenosine deaminase (ADA) deficiency, can be treated with the missing ADA enzyme. The first gene therapies used in humans were developed for ADA and X-linked forms of SCID, Puck said, and they are considered curative. Because most SCID cases are sporadic, newborn screening would be needed to identify infants prior to them developing infectious complications, Puck said, given that survival is compromised by infections at the time of the gene therapy treatment (Pai et al., 2014).

A specific form of SCID caused by the recessive mutation *DCLRE-1CY192X* in the Artemis gene[2] occurs at a higher rate in the Navajo and closely related Apache tribes of Native Americans. This genetic variant was present in the survivors of the 1864 "Long Walk," which killed 90 percent of the people who started the forced resettlement journey from Arizona to New Mexico, thus creating a genetic bottleneck that is thought to have increased the population incidence of this recessive gene. It is estimated that 1 in 2,000 Navajo and Apache infants have this form of SCID, Puck said.

In an unpublished study conducted at the University of California, San Francisco, by Morton Cowan, a small group of Navajo SCID patients were treated with a bone marrow transplant and followed for 24 years. Those individuals, diagnosed very early in life because they had an affected sibling, had a higher survival rate than individuals who were diagnosed because of infections, Puck said. Researchers have since discovered a blood-borne biomarker for SCID called T-cell receptor excision circles, which serves as a marker of T-cell maturation. Today, screening for SCID is part of the Recommended Uniform Screening Panel, a list of disorders that the Secretary of the Department of Health and Human Services encourages states to test for as part of newborn screening programs. However, when Puck and her colleagues undertook a SCID screening study in Navajos in 2009, this method was relatively new, and there was quite a bit of distrust among the Navajo based on past exploitation by population genetics researchers, Puck said. In fact, the Navajo institutional review board initially prohibited genetic testing on study samples and required written, face-to-face consent. Nonetheless, in 2011, after 1,800 research samples were collected and analyzed, the test was adopted reservation-wide as the standard of care.

Recent studies conducted by the Primary Immune Deficiency Treatment Consortium demonstrated that the survival rate after receiving a donor transplant depends on the exact SCID genotype, with the Artemis genotype having the worst survival rate, likely because the genetic defect results in impaired DNA repair, which is not isolated to the immune system (Haddad et al., 2018). This form of SCID is the most difficult to treat with allogeneic bone marrow cell transplant, Puck said, and autologous gene therapy may be a better approach. In collaboration with Scott McIvor at the University of Minnesota, Puck and her colleagues created a self-inactivating lentiviral vector containing the human *DCLRE1C* promoter, and as of October 2019 her group used that vector to treat four newly diagnosed infants and three older children with SCID who had been previously transplanted but developed insufficient immunity. Two of the infants and two of the older children were Navajo. Newborn screening will be a critical element of this

---

[2]The Artemis protein is involved in V(D)J recombination, a process important for the development and maturation of T and B cells.

trial going forward, Puck said, because it provides an unbiased population-level ability to make an early diagnosis, which in turn promotes fair access to treatment.

In closing, Puck said that the Navajos now embrace SCID screening and early treatment, though achieving optimal outcomes is challenged by distance from medical facilities, poverty, and social difficulties. Having a network of trusted local physicians has been critical to this effort, Puck said, and she and her team travel to the reservation annually to hold SCID clinics. It is important to note that the entire therapeutic process for SCID can be extremely stressful for Navajo families who have to remain with their child for upward of 3 months as the child develops his or her own T cells.

THE CHALLENGES OF USING GENE THERAPY TO TREAT DUCHENNE MUSCULAR DYSTROPHY

As Richard Finkel noted in the first panel session, DMD is an X chromosome–linked childhood genetic disease. DMD most often affects boys, although in rare cases girls can develop a milder form of the condition (MDA, 2020). Pat Furlong explained that about 30 percent of cases of DMD are due to random spontaneous mutations in which there is no family history of DMD. Other families find out they are carriers of a DMD causative genetic variant after they have had children. The standard of care for individuals with DMD has evolved over the years, with corticosteroid treatment now enabling them to walk until they are 10 to 13 years old, but most affected children still lose mobility in their arms by age 16 or 17, require noninvasive ventilation in their late teens, and die at an average age of 28.

Dystrophin, the gene responsible for DMD, is one of the largest genes in the human genome and was first cloned in 1986 (Monaco et al., 1986). Researchers have identified more than 1,000 mutations in the dystrophin gene that result in DMD. When the protein product of dystrophin was identified in 1987, Furlong said, many investigators were confident that gene therapy for DMD would be straightforward. However, she continued, more than 30 years later clinical trials for a gene-based therapy for DMD are just beginning. The trials are using a viral vector that delivers a small piece of the dystrophin gene because the entire gene is too large to deliver successfully with existing vectors.

Parents who have been recruited to put their children in trials often recall being shown an image of a 65-year-old man with DMD playing tennis, Furlong said. This individual is asymptomatic and provided the rationale for researchers to develop a synthetic, shortened version of dystrophin. The near-universal response when parents see this man's image, she said, is a desire to access this treatment for their children. However, she added, what they may not be told is that this man was not given the gene therapy construct, known as a microdystrophin, but instead has had this microdystrophin existing naturally in his genome since birth. Nonetheless, the clinical trial has started to recruit 4- to 7-year-olds. These early trials require the child and a parent to stay at the clinical site for approximately 30 days after treatment, Furlong said. Parents are worried about the age restrictions, especially if their children are slightly older or younger than the target age range, Furlong said. Parents also worry about protecting their children from environmental exposures that might trigger an immune response to the viral vector if and when they are accepted into a trial, she explained.

The requirement to stay at the clinical site means that families without resources or support at home or who have employers who may not be enthusiastic about granting 30 days of leave are unlikely to participate in the trial. Furlong said she has seen families move to be near a clinical site or take out second mortgages on their homes to pay for the indirect costs associated with participating in a gene therapy clinical trial. The current informed consent process is not very informative, Furlong said, and families may not even realize that by agreeing to have their child participate in a gene therapy trial, they are opting out of every one of the other 27 active clinical trials taking place in the DMD space.

Aside from worries about the muscle biopsies that are done under anesthesia and the doubling of the steroid doses that comes with getting the therapy, another common parental concern is whether the child is receiving the experimental treatment or is part of the control group that will eventually receive the active therapy once the trial is over. Furlong also said that in some cases the elevated steroid dose results in negative side effects and behavioral issues in the children. All of these factors, she said, create a large burden on families while also giving them hope.

One concern brought up by Furlong involves muscle turnover in those children treated with gene therapy. Because it is unclear if children can be re-dosed with gene therapy, she asked, will cases of teenage-onset DMD appear? She said that it is important to think about when to deliver subsequent doses of the gene therapy, given that waiting until older boys start showing signs means that there will be parts of their body subject to irreparable damage from which their bodies cannot recover.

A final issue Furlong mentioned was the question of what to tell the children who participate in these clinical trials. She recalled one boy who was in the trial but not showing improvement, and he started acting out likely because of his disappointment that the "magic medicine" was not working as well as everyone had hoped. Information that is communicated to children and families involved in pediatric gene therapy trials is important because they look forward to these types of therapeutic opportunities, Furlong said, but the trials come with many complicated issues.

PATIENT AND FAMILY PERSPECTIVES

Contreras, whose family lives in Chile, has two sons with DMD and her older son, 5-year-old Franco, is enrolled in the microdystrophin gene therapy clinical trial. She and her husband learned about gene therapy and clinical trials for DMD after months of intensive research, which led them to contact the organizers of three clinical trials. One researcher got back in touch with the Contreras family and told them that the trials were not accepting international patients. The result was that the family secured visas that allowed them to move to the United States and find work. "We are so grateful, and at the same time very aware of all of the families around the world, but also within the United States, that just cannot afford the direct and indirect costs of participating in a gene therapy clinical trial," she said.

One concern of Contreras and her husband was that their son would receive a placebo, a risk they were willing to take. What was not acceptable to them was the possibility that their son would receive a suboptimal dose of the therapy, so they chose to prioritize participating in the clinical trial that did not include a dose escalation component. After Franco was accepted into a trial, the family was told to keep their younger son Julián away from Franco for the next 30 days so that he would not be exposed to the viral vector, develop immunity to it, and then be ineligible for accessing gene therapy in the future. As a result, her husband Pablo took a 24-hour, round-trip journey from Columbus, Ohio, to Santiago, Chile, to take Julián back and made it to Ohio in time for Franco's infusion. A few days later, Pablo returned to Chile while María stayed in Columbus with Franco.

Contreras said that for her family, one of the most sensitive ethical issues is a lack of a sibling protocol. "We are giving Franco an opportunity that at this point we are not sure we will be able to provide to Julián," she said. For pediatric incurable diseases such as DMD, the need for a sibling protocol is urgent, she said. Other needs, Contreras said, include an expedited regulatory process and improved trial accessibility for patients in early and advanced phases of the disease, for international populations, for boys and girls, and for families that cannot afford to participate in clinical trials. Trial design could be improved by the development of innovative protocols that minimize placebo arms and use natural history studies, master protocols that may combine different therapeutic approaches, and the increased involvement of patients and families in protocol design. "Our voices should be heard not only when we say yes and sign the consent form, but throughout the process," she said in closing.

Another perspective on these issues came from Samuels, a participant in a gene therapy clinical trial for sickle cell disease. Diagnosed at age 2, her symptoms grew progressively worse, and by the time she was 7 she experienced her first aplastic anemia crisis, which occurs when bone marrow does not produce enough red blood cells. At 13 years old, Samuels suffered a transient ischemic attack, which for months presented as a mild stroke that affected the left side of her face and arms. Soon after, the pain associated with her disease became severe enough that by the time she was a sophomore in high school, she was being home schooled so that she could continue to get an education while being treated with high doses of opioids, monthly blood transfusions, and nightly 10-hour infusions of deferoxamine mesylate to prevent the iron toxicity related to those blood infusions.

Samuels detailed more of the medical emergencies she suffered over the years and noted that she got married in 2008 and had an ectopic pregnancy that triggered another crisis in 2011. In 2015, she was told that liver dialysis would be the next step, which set her off on a persistent search for a clinical trial to join. That persistence paid off, and she enrolled in the NHLBI trial using an autologous gene therapy transplant rather than requiring a matched donor bone marrow transplant.

The gene therapy process that Tisdale and his colleagues laid out for her in great detail, both in writing and verbally, was almost too much to take in for her and her family, Samuels said. "I was contemplating signing up for something that would put my body through high doses of chemo, make me menopausal before the age of 40, take months in a hospital, and agree to at least 3 years of monitoring, and when I considered those things and what I had already gone through, this to me was a godsend," she explained. "It took a year for me to convince my family of that fact, but I got them to see that as well."

When Samuels went to the clinical center at NIH in March 2018 for the gene therapy, she did not know what to expect, she said, and it was difficult to keep her emotions in check. However, she said, being surrounded daily by doctors, nurses, nutritionists, and other members of the care team made it a bit easier to trust the process, despite all of the ongoing challenges. It also helped to be able to call people who had gone through the debilitating chemotherapy process before, Samuels said. On the day of the workshop, which took place almost 2 years after the gene therapy administration, Samuels reported that she no longer experiences daily pain, no longer needs narcotics to get out of bed, and has not needed a blood transfusion since August 2018. Today, she said, she makes it a point to "live out loud," because she was unable to do so for such a long time. "I came here to maintain my hope in the health and rebirth of what science is doing today," she said in closing.

Bartek began his short presentation by explaining that there is no current gene therapy clinical trial for Friedreich's ataxia, a genetic neuromuscular disorder, although there are groups currently advancing gene therapy research programs for this disease. The issue of developing gene therapies for rare diseases was the focus of a 2-day workshop held in 2018[3] that was sponsored by the National Center for Advancing Translational Sciences (NCATS) and FDA's Office of Tissues and Advanced Therapies. "For 2 days, we heard academic and industry investigators talk about the issues that were confounding their gene therapy trials," Bartek said.

From those presentations, he said, it was clear that while the successes achieved differed from trial to trial, there were several shared challenges. He compiled a list of five to six issues that were confounding all of these investigations, and after sharing this list with the NCATS leadership, a new program was created under the auspices of the Cures Acceleration Network Review Board to develop advanced technology platform solutions to address the issues he had identified.

Turning to the family perspective on gene therapy clinical trials, Bartek said that safety is a concern, but given that there are no approved treatments for many of these diseases, families are often willing to take substantial risks. Perhaps the gravest concern of families is whether their loved ones will receive a therapeutic dose of the investigational agent. In his opinion, Bartek said, the paradigm of starting trials in adults or only symptomatic patients to prove safety has to change, especially because time is of the essence for pediatric patients; similarly, he said, the assumption that gene therapy is to be a "one-and-done" treatment also must change. "Can we either use different vectors or different routes of administration so that over time we can get a second dose?" he asked. He also posed several other questions, including

- Are there alternatives to a placebo in a clinical trial?
- Is it possible to work around exclusion from a trial based on a previous exposure to these viral vectors?
- Is it possible to know in advance how therapeutic a gene therapy will be?
- Can we educate the patient and the family about expectations?
- How long will it take the field to get to these particular rare diseases?

---

[3]The August 2018 workshop, The Growing Promise of Gene Therapy Approaches to Rare Diseases, was jointly sponsored by the National Center for Advancing Translational Sciences and the Food and Drug Administration's Center for Biologics Evaluation and Research. More information about the workshop and the agenda can be found at https://events-support.com/events/NCATS_Gene_Therapy_2018 (accessed February 19, 2020).

Regarding the last question, Bartek said that there are some 7,000 rare genetic diseases and that the current pace of development is far too slow to treat a meaningful number of these diseases in the foreseeable future.

One recommendation Bartek made was for the field to support the creation of a common manufacturing facility that would have capacity to provide sufficient material for a small Phase 1 clinical trial led by academic investigators rather than leaving very early investigations to a pharmaceutical company that would have to invest $200 million in a manufacturing facility before even starting a clinical development program. Another recommendation from Bartek was for NCATS and FDA to collaborate on developing a standardized clinical trial design that would be widely applicable to rare diseases. In conclusion, Bartek said, it is important that novel gene therapies be fairly priced in order to promote equitable access for patients and sustainable reimbursement for payers.

DISCUSSION

Following the presentations, all of the speakers participated in a moderated panel discussion that included questions from the audience. Points raised in this discussion period primarily centered on the development of educational materials for patients and families and issues with the informed consent process.

Patient- and Family-Centered Educational Materials and Access to Statisticians

Educational materials about new technologies such as CRISPR/Cas-9, zinc finger nucleases, and other gene-editing techniques would be useful in helping patients and families understand the clinical process, one workshop participant said. NIH is developing such materials to make the process more understandable for patients and their families, Tisdale responded. The reason that his team uses CRISPR/Cas-9 instead of some of the other gene-editing techniques has to do with patents and ready access to the technology, he said. The participant went on to ask the two NIH speakers why their gene therapy trial stopped using the hydroxyurea treatment, which can reduce the number of pain episodes substantially. Tisdale answered that hydroxyurea also reduces the number of bone marrow stem cells that can be harvested from patients, which would reduce the likelihood of reaching the therapeutic target dose. Thus, in order to harvest sufficient quantities of bone marrow stem cells from patients, hydroxyurea treatments stop and exchange transfusions are used instead, Tisdale said, as a way to yield a better product that is less prone to downstream complications.

A workshop participant asked if any of the patients or family members on the panel had a chance to discuss concerns with statisticians involved with a clinical trial before or during enrollment. Samuels said no, but said she thought that might be a good option in the future. Bartek said that the Friedreich's Ataxia Research Alliance has had tremendous access to the statistical community, including enlisting statisticians to help fortify and analyze the organization's natural history database. Recently, in collaboration with FDA and the National Organization for Rare Disorders, his organization has populated its natural history database by adding placebo arm data from clinical trials with help from statisticians. Furlong added that Parent Project Muscular Dystrophy has been working with the Critical Path Institute to develop a disease progression model.

The Informed Consent Process

Regarding informed consent, Cho said that many patients and families are experts in their own diseases and understand the risks and benefits of participating in a clinical trial. At the same time, she said, empirical studies have shown that while people may understand that there are risks of death and severe morbidity from participating in clinical trials, the issue is the extent to which individuals believe that they are in the population that is going to be subject to those risks. Given the difficulty that people have of reconciling the existence of risks in clinical trials with their beliefs about their chances for successful outcomes in those trials, she asked if the panelists had any suggestions for overcoming that cognitive dissonance. A gene therapy consent form can be more than 20 pages of tiny, single-spaced type, making it nearly impossible to explain everything in it in one sitting, Puck said, let alone allow the patient to take in and process all of that information. She suggested that it would be a good idea to have many conversations about participating in gene therapy clinical trials and to let people know that they maintain control over stopping their participation right up to the moment they are infused with the treatment, at which point they need to be partners with the research team going forward. "I think communication, trust, and partnership do not develop over one consent form," Puck said. Instead, it takes days or weeks, at least, to develop this sort of relationship, she said.

Fitzhugh agreed with Puck and said she asks patients and families to take the consent form home, read it on their own schedule, and write down any questions they have. She also counsels them to talk to their own family physicians and to reach out to other patients. Samuels said that she received the consent form 1 year before she decided to sign it, giving her time to pore over the document and come to her own conclusions. In addition, she said, she had had several conversations with the research team nurses and a meeting with family and friends before she signed the form.

The process should shift from a consent form as a timepoint event to a consent process, Contreras said, and the research teams should always suggest reaching out to other patients who have gone through the procedure. In the case of her son Franco, she said, the family was asked to re-consent to a change in the protocol that would double the steroid dose after receiving the therapeutic agent. "I would have appreciated if I had received more information from the sponsors and the medical team as to why these changes were made and what the rationale was for making them," she said. Furlong suggested that it might be helpful if there were a summary page preceding the actual consent form that would refer to the most important pieces of information. Similarly, for re-consent, the front page could point to the exact spot in the original consent form to which proposed changes apply.

Panelists were asked if they had ever encountered cases where parents and children were at odds over signing the consent form. Furlong said that typically young boys with DMD do what their parents say, and Puck said that the children she has worked with and who are old enough cognitively to understand the process have been extremely enthusiastic about participating in a clinical trial, even after learning that the procedure may not work for them.

4

Developing Endpoints for
Gene Therapy Clinical Trials

Important Points Highlighted by Individual Speakers

- Long-term or potentially irreversible effects of gene therapy treatments leave little room for uncertainty about their end-point performance and require increased vigilance concerning the validity and accuracy of endpoint measurement. (Lapteva)
- Mechanistically agnostic endpoints reflective of common pathogenic pathways may not be sufficient in gene therapy clinical trials. Due to the increased availability of genetic screening, early diagnosis, and advanced laboratory testing, there has been a shift toward using surrogate and clinical endpoints that reflect early disease manifestations. (Lapteva)
- It can be challenging to differentiate between the effects of a standard-of-care therapy versus an experimental gene therapy. In the case of Pompe disease, researchers plan to enroll patients who are stably treated with the standard of care in a gene therapy trial, with the expectation that any improvements in muscle function can be attributed to the gene therapy. Examining baseline levels and patient history is also important as a way to determine if changes in clinical outcomes are due to the experimental therapy. (Koeberl)
- The multi-luminance mobility test (MLMT) was developed as a clinically meaningful endpoint for patients with a form of congenital retinal dystrophy. The MLMT can differentiate subjects

---

with low vision from those with normal vision, detect changes in clinically meaningful visual function over time, and identify a wide range of performance characteristics among the visually impaired. In the case of retinal disorders, the MLMT was preferred as an endpoint over pupillometry because improvements in functional vision are very meaningful to patients. (Maguire)

- There is a great deal of phenotypic diversity among patients with sickle cell disease, which makes the identification of clinically meaningful endpoints very challenging. There is a need for a national registry for sickle cell disease patients as a way to collect natural history data and develop reliable and clinically meaningful endpoints. (Kanter)
- Investigators will need to monitor gene therapy recipients over the long term to see if the therapies provide long-term disease management or a cure and to figure out how to make this type of therapy available, affordable, and universal. (Kanter)

The third workshop panel explored the successes with and challenges to accurately measuring clinical endpoints and outcomes for gene-based therapies and moving products through the translational pathway. Larissa Lapteva, the associate director in the Division of Clinical Evaluation, Pharmacology, and Toxicology, Office of Tissues and Advanced Therapies, Center for Biologics Evaluation and Research at FDA, moderated the session. She noted in her introductory remarks that for any clinical development program with a novel therapeutic product, the choice of the primary endpoint for a clinical trial intended to demonstrate substantial evidence of that product or that agent's effectiveness can be the most vulnerable part of the entire development program. This can either unite all of the elements of that development or make the product nonviable, she said. Lapteva also described some of the important concepts regarding endpoints and outcomes in clinical trials. Dwight Koeberl, a professor of pediatrics and molecular genetics and microbiology in the Department of Pediatrics at Duke University and the medical director of the Duke University Health System Biochemical Genetics Laboratory, discussed endpoints for clinical trials in Pompe disease; Albert Maguire, a professor of ophthalmology at the Hospital of the University of Pennsylvania and the Presbyterian Medical Center of Philadelphia, discussed clinical endpoints for a Phase 3 inherited retinal dystrophy gene therapy trial; and Julie Kanter, an associate professor of hematology and oncology at the University of Alabama at Birmingham School of Medicine, discussed her work determining optimal endpoints for gene therapy trials in sickle cell disease.

DEVELOPING ENDPOINTS FOR CLINICAL TRIALS

The concept of "substantial evidence of effectiveness" for human drugs and biological products has been defined and codified in the Code of Federal Regulations and is described and discussed in many FDA guidance documents, Lapteva said. Briefly, she explained that FDA requires two adequate and well-controlled clinical trials for most diseases, though in some cases—for example, in rare diseases where a second trial might not be feasible or ethical—FDA will accept one adequate and well-controlled trial with supportive confirmatory evidence.

In the traditional regulatory approval pathway, the endpoints used in the trials that are intended to demonstrate the product's evidence of effectiveness would be clinical endpoints that directly measure clinical benefit or surrogate endpoints that have been validated to predict clinical benefit.[1] A second pathway, accelerated approval, has been around since the 1990s and is typically reserved for serious and, often, rare diseases for which there are no available treatments. Accelerated approval has been used in cases where the disease course may be prolonged and an extended period would be needed to observe clinical benefit.[2] In order to make development feasible and also improve access to care for those who need it, accelerated approval allows for the use of surrogate endpoints that predict clinical benefit with reasonable likelihood, Lapteva said.

Clinical outcomes, when used as endpoints, directly measure clinical benefit, which FDA views as how a patient feels, functions, or survives, Lapteva said. Surrogate endpoints (which may be laboratory parameters) can be measured earlier than clinical outcomes, but their use in trials should be supported by an ability to predict clinical benefit. For years the term "surrogate endpoint" was largely misunderstood and used interchangeably with other similar terms, confusing its meaning, Lapteva said, so FDA and NIH collaborated on developing the Biomarkers, EndpointS, and other Tools (BEST) resource, which was published in 2015.[3] According to BEST, surrogate endpoints can be divided into the following summary categories:

---

[1]For FDA guidance on clinical trial endpoints, see https://www.fda.gov/regulatory-information/search-fda-guidance-documents/clinical-trial-endpoints-approval-cancer-drugs-and-biologics (accessed January 13, 2020).

[2]For FDA guidance on expedited programs for serious conditions, see https://www.fda.gov/regulatory-information/search-fda-guidance-documents/expedited-programs-serious-conditions-drugs-and-biologics (accessed January 13, 2020).

[3]Additional information on the Biomarkers, EndpointS, and other Tools resource is available at https://www.ncbi.nlm.nih.gov/books/NBK338448 (accessed January 13, 2020).

- **Validated surrogate endpoints** are those supported by a clear mechanistic rational as well as by clinical data providing evidence that the surrogate endpoint predicts a specific clinical benefit.
- **Reasonably likely surrogate endpoints** are supported by a strong mechanistic or epidemiologic rationale but lack adequate clinical data showing that the surrogate endpoint will predict a specific clinical benefit.
- **Candidate surrogate endpoints** are still under evaluation as to how they may predict clinical benefit.

FDA, Lapteva said, has posted lists of endpoints used in traditional and accelerated approvals of drugs and biological products.[4] In the case of gene therapies under development, FDA recognizes that for many diseases for which gene therapies may be beneficial (i.e., rare genetic diseases), there are no reliable clinical or surrogate endpoints, particularly endpoints reflective of early disease manifestations. In those cases, she said, investigators need to develop novel endpoints.

In closing, Lapteva listed some points to consider in choosing endpoints for clinical trials with gene therapies:

- The possibility of long-term or potentially irreversible effects of gene therapy treatments leaves little room for uncertainty about endpoint performance at the stage of study design and requires increased vigilance concerning the validity and accuracy of endpoint measurements during the study.
- Endpoints reflective of common pathogenic pathways, but mechanistically agnostic to the target disease or condition, may not be sufficiently sensitive in gene therapy clinical trials. Indeed, the increased availability of genetic screening, early diagnosis, and advanced laboratory testing has shifted the demand toward surrogate and clinical endpoints reflective of early disease manifestations, while the identification of genetic defects associated with poorly characterized phenotypes has increased the need for novel clinical endpoints.
- In addition to finding disease-specific surrogate endpoints, there may be an opportunity to identify and validate surrogate endpoints along the universal pathway of gene transcription, transgene protein synthesis and levels, functional activity, and clearance. The

---

[4]Additional information is available at https://www.fda.gov/drugs/development-resources/table-surrogate-endpoints-were-basis-drug-approval-or-licensure (accessed December 11, 2019) and https://www.fda.gov/drugs/development-resources/clinical-outcome-assessment-compendium (accessed December 11, 2019).

principles of such endpoint identification and validation may be applicable to multiple diseases and different types of gene therapy products.

ENDPOINTS FOR GENE THERAPY CLINICAL TRIALS IN POMPE DISEASE

Focusing in on clinical endpoints for a specific condition, Koeberl began his presentation by giving a brief background on Pompe disease. Pompe disease, or glycogen storage disease type II, is caused by a deficiency of the enzyme acid alpha-glucosidase (GAA) in skeletal muscle and heart. It can be treated successfully by giving patients GAA, which is taken up by a receptor in muscle and heart cells. Enzyme replacement therapy is the standard of care for the disease; by contrast, the approach that Koeberl and his colleagues have taken is to create a recombinant AAV8 vector to deliver the GAA gene to the liver, where it can produce high levels of GAA that enters into blood circulation and eventually travels to the heart and muscle cells, correcting the GAA deficiency.

The primary advantage of this liver-specific expression, Koeberl explained, is that it suppresses the production of antibodies against GAA, which can interfere with the current GAA enzyme replacement therapy.[5] Other potential advantages of a gene therapy approach versus enzyme replacement therapy that have been identified from preclinical studies include sustained levels of GAA in blood, an increased uptake of GAA by muscle, a more complete correction of the enzymatic deficit, potentially decreased mortality, and a one-time dose of the gene therapy vector versus required injections of GAA every 1 to 2 weeks (Bond et al., 2019). Experiments in mice showed that GAA levels in the liver, heart, diaphragm, and quadriceps increased more in the mice that received one dose of gene therapy than in mice that received four injections of the enzyme (Han et al., 2017, 2019). Glycogen content, however, is a more sensitive measure of biochemical correction, and both treatments significantly decreased the amount of glycogen in the heart and diaphragm.

Koeberl discussed how his group chose the endpoints for its clinical trial from the multiple endpoints that have already been developed for Pompe disease. One of the challenges in developing a standalone gene therapy for the disease, he said, is having to manage the interactions between the standard-of-care treatment and the gene therapy because withholding standard of care in the early phases of disease would be unethical. "We

---

[5]The liver-targeted gene therapy delivery and expression of GAA induces immune tolerance by suppressing regulatory T cells.

have to consider that when we are designing endpoints and when we are collecting data," Koeberl said.

Touching on all of the available endpoints and outcomes for Pompe disease, Koeberl briefly described a recent Phase 1/2 clinical trial of clenbuterol (Koeberl et al., 2018). The intent of this study was to gain a better understanding of how patients who received clenbuterol improved from baseline over time in terms of endpoints such as the 6-minute walk test, pulmonary function tests, and a muscle biopsy. Switching gears back to gene therapy approaches for Pompe disease, Koeberl discussed an ongoing Phase 1 trial of the AAV8 vector, in which safety is the primary endpoint. Safety in this trial is being evaluated by the incidence of adverse events and through monitoring clinical laboratory abnormalities, he said. Secondary endpoints include muscle function and pulmonary function tests, GAA activity and glycogen content in muscle biopsies, antibody formation, a urinary biomarker, and serum levels of GAA, the last of which Koeberl characterized as "very exploratory." Except for the last endpoint, each of the secondary endpoints was validated in the earlier clinical trial with clenbuterol, with two markers of muscle and pulmonary function suitable for using in a regulatory submission, he said (Koeberl et al., 2018).

On the issue of how to tease apart the effects of standard of care and gene therapy, Koeberl explained that standard of care will stabilize muscle function, but further improvements will decline after the first couple of years of therapy (Harlaar et al., 2019). Therefore, the plan will be to enroll stably treated patients, which will make it possible to credit any improvement in muscle function to gene therapy, not enzyme replacement therapy. Koeberl noted, however, that for individuals, it is important to look at baseline levels and history before attributing improvements to gene therapy because someone who has been treated with enzyme replacement therapy for a long time may have a number of variables to consider. GAA levels also fluctuate during enzyme replacement therapy, he said, so the timing of a muscle biopsy relative to treatments with enzyme replacement therapy is important. It will also be necessary to stop standard of care at some point to demonstrate that gene therapy can serve as a standalone treatment, which will require well-designed criteria for withdrawing standard of care as well as reinstituting it if needed. Muscle glycogen content could be a good surrogate endpoint, once validated, Koeberl said, given that Pompe disease is a glycogen storage disease with glycogen accumulation being integral to disease pathogenesis.

A NOVEL OUTCOME MEASURE FOR GENE THERAPY
FOR A FORM OF CONGENITAL BLINDNESS

The discussion on developing endpoints was continued by Maguire, who spoke about a novel outcome measure for Leber congenital amaurosis, a rare, autosomal recessive form of congenital retinal dystrophy that causes blindness. This condition results from lack-of-function mutations in the *RPE65* gene as described in Katherine High's earlier presentation. Humans and affected animals—there are naturally occurring dog models of this disease—with these mutations have early-onset blindness, abnormal eye movements, and flat electrical responses to light stimulation, Maguire said. Before gene therapy, there was no treatment for the disorder. As High noted in her presentation, gene therapy with an AAV vector carrying the wild-type *RPE65* gene restored some vision to affected individuals.

For the Phase 1 trial of the AAV.hRPE65v2 gene therapy, Maguire and his colleagues used pupillometry, which provided objective evidence for improved function as an outcome measure. Maguire explained that pupillary light reflex is restored in retina exposed to the gene therapy construct and not in the uninjected, or contralateral, retina (Maguire et al., 2008, 2009). The issue with using this objective test for the FDA Phase 3 trial, Maguire said, was that pupillometry was not considered a clinically meaningful outcome. As one FDA reviewer put it, patients care about vision, not about their pupils, a sentiment with which Maguire agreed.

At the time, he said, there was no recognized outcome measure considered clinically meaningful, except for one surrogate endpoint: three lines of improvement on an eye chart. While some patients showed an improvement in visual acuity, which is central vision, the main improvement with the AAV.hRPE65v2 gene therapy is mediated by rod photoreceptors, which are involved in peripheral vision and night vision, he explained. The problem was that there was no test for this type of vision that satisfied the clinically meaningful, clinically significant mandate.

In the Phase 1/2 trial, Maguire's team looked at mobility testing, which is essentially the ability to navigate an obstacle course in a certain amount of time, as an exploratory endpoint. An initial test of this endpoint showed that children who received the gene therapy were able to go through the course much more quickly when using their injected eye than when using their uninjected eye (Maguire et al., 2009). A more advanced form of this test measured the time to complete the obstacle course at seven different light levels ranging from 1 lux to 400 lux. FDA suggested that this test could be a good outcome measure and essentially assigned Maguire and his colleagues the task of creating a new outcome measure based on this framework. "FDA provided some excellent feedback on developing this into a standardized, statistically rigorous test that would satisfy the clinically meaningful mandate," Maguire said.

The resulting MLMT is a novel metric that measures the speed and accuracy with which a subject can ambulate independently under different ambient light conditions. Maguire and his team built 12 obstacle courses, the choice of which was randomized for each run at a specific light level corresponding to various light conditions encountered during daily living (Russell et al., 2017). For example, a moonless summer night would be 1 lux of intensity, an outdoor train station at night would be 50 lux, and a bright office building would be 400 lux. Subjects were dark-adapted for 40 minutes and then asked to navigate a course as quickly as possible with the fewest errors possible, Maguire said, adding that FDA helped his team develop the test to be rigorous, objective, and reproducible. Each patient video was reviewed and graded by two examiners, who were blind as to whether the test was performed pre- or post-treatment, Maguire said.

A validation study of the MLMT showed that its results correlated with measures of visual acuity and visual field. Normal-sighted subjects all passed the test (with regard to time and accuracy) at all light levels (Chung et al., 2018). None of the individuals with inherited retinal disease improved from baseline to year 1, and 28.5 percent of the subjects declined in performance over 1 year.

In the Phase 3 trial that FDA approved, Maguire said, the MLMT provided clear evidence for a statistically significant improvement in visual function for patients receiving gene therapy (Chung et al., 2018). In addition, he said, the results of this test correlated well with measures of visual function such as sensitivity, which is the ability to perceive different ambient light levels, and for two different measures of visual field.

In summary, Maguire said, the MLMT is a novel test that was developed to provide a primary outcome measure for subjects receiving investigational products for inherited retinal dystrophies resulting in reduced retinal sensitivity and visual field. Its essential features include the ability to differentiate low-vision subjects from normal subjects, to detect changes in clinically meaningful visual function over time, and to identify a wide range of performance characteristics among the visually impaired.

DETERMINING OPTIMAL ENDPOINTS FOR GENE THERAPY IN SICKLE CELL DISEASE

Developing endpoints for sickle cell disease has long been a challenge for the field and was recently the focus of a workshop hosted by the

American Society of Hematology and FDA, Kanter said.[6] One reason it has been difficult to develop clinical endpoints is because there is a large amount of phenotypic diversity associated with the disease, which is not necessarily accounted for by hemoglobin genotypes, she said. "While clinical patterns exist, each individual with sickle cell disease is unique and may have a unique clinical course," Kanter said.

The one hallmark feature of sickle cell disease, she said, is pain, the primary reason why individuals with this disease will encounter medical specialists throughout their lives. The consequence with the most impact, however, is death. While childhood mortality has improved significantly since the 1970s, when more than 10 percent of children with the sickle cell mutation died by age 4, little progress has occurred regarding adult mortality, with sickle cell patients dying, on average, in their early 40s (Paulukonis et al., 2016; Quinn et al., 2010).

One of the challenges facing researchers working on new treatments for sickle cell disease, Kanter said, is that there is no national registry of patients even though there are more than 100,000 individuals with sickle cell disease in the United States alone. The lack of a national registry makes it hard to conduct natural history studies, she said, as well as making it difficult to determine optimal endpoints for clinical trials.

Current therapies, Kanter said, include small molecule drugs (e.g., hydroxyurea, L-glutamine), blood transfusions, and palliative pain management. Due primarily to the wide disparity in benefits and side effects, none of these therapies are broadly accepted. Stem cell transplants, as Courtney Fitzhugh described in her earlier presentation, can cure sickle cell disease and are particularly promising for children with matched related donors; the risk versus benefit for adults is improving as well, and early studies paint an optimistic picture for improved outcomes and quality of life (Aslam et al., 2018). Stem cell transplants do come with the risk of GVHD and can require immune suppressive medication over the long term. There is also the risk of a late rejection of the transplant. Gene therapy, Kanter said, would circumvent the need to find a matched donor; it can take the form of either adding a new gene that produces normally functioning hemoglobin or gene editing, which would correct the mutation in the body.

The most commonly used primary endpoint has been pain severity during a vaso-occlusive crisis, but, as Kanter pointed out, pain is subjective and

---

[6]Following the workshop, in December 2019, two publications that discuss the findings from the American Society of Hematology and FDA meeting were released. The first paper covers patient-reported outcomes, pain, and issues with the brain and can be found at https://ashpublications.org/bloodadvances/article/3/23/3982/429244 (accessed January 26, 2020). The second paper that explores renal and cardiopulmonary endpoints along with a measurement of the cure and a discussion of low-resource settings can be found at https://ashpublications.org/bloodadvances/article/3/23/4002/429243 (accessed January 26, 2020).

can have many causes having nothing to do with sickle cell disease. Various biologic endpoints have been proposed, but none have been validated in sickle cell disease, and the same is true for biologic predictors of disease severity. "We cannot identify, when a person is born with sickle cell disease, if it will be severe, if they will have frequent pain crises and be in the hospital frequently, or even if the disease will not manifest itself until the individual is a young adult," Kanter said.

There was hope that the presence of fetal hemoglobin might predict individuals who will have an easier disease course, but studies have found that many adults with persistent fetal hemoglobin have all of the same complications as those without persistent fetal hemoglobin, even though the disease appears 10 to 20 years later in those with persistent fetal hemoglobin. Total hemoglobin does seem to correlate with some disease-specific mortality measures, such as renal dysfunction and stroke, Kanter said, but it is unclear if altering an individual's total hemoglobin prior to disease manifestation will change the disease course.

The outcomes of stem cell transplants have demonstrated something important, Kanter said, and have shown that sufficient engraftment of donor stem cells leads to curative therapy. These studies have also provided evidence that stem cell transplants are successful when they result in non-sickle hemoglobin engraftment accounting for at least 50 percent of total hemoglobin production (produced from as little as 20 percent of the stem cells in patients with mixed chimerism). With gene therapy, she explained, the goal is to have pancellular expression, where every bone marrow cell expresses both non-sickle (hemoglobin A or F) and sickle cell hemoglobin. When red blood cells express both forms of hemoglobin, the normal hemoglobin can outcompete the sickled form resulting in red blood cells with a normal (or near normal) shape. Incomplete transfection or subtherapeutic doses that do not result in pancellular expression would allow for the formation of some red blood cells with only the mutant hemoglobin, which would cause sickling and clinical complications.

Work done with bluebird bio (a biotechnology company based in Massachusetts), using a vector that delivers a functional adult hemoglobin gene rather than a fetal hemoglobin gene, has shown that the vector copy number (the average number of gene therapy vectors delivered to a sample of blood stem cells), the percentage of stem cells that have been transduced or have received a gene therapy vector, and cell dose (the amount of a patient's own blood stem cells returned to the patient after transduction was delivered) correlate well with the quantity of hemoglobin those cells produce. The vector copy number can predict how much novel therapeutic hemoglobin the patient will make, Kanter said. She noted, too, that clinical studies have shown that over time the amount of healthy hemoglobin increases because those cells outlive the sickled hemoglobin-containing cells.

While clinical results so far have been encouraging, it will be important to determine how individuals receiving gene-based therapy do over the long term regarding resolution of vaso-occlusive pain, decrease in stroke risk, and stabilization of organ dysfunction. There are safety concerns with gene therapies, Kanter noted, including insertional oncogenesis and a lack of sustainable protein production. There might also be off-target effects that will be difficult to identify, and novel mutations may occur. Research needs to determine the stopping points at which an investigation would end with poor outcomes and identify measures to define success that will be accepted by FDA and other regulatory agencies, she said. Currently, there are no stopping guidelines; however, Kanter said, as more information is gathered, there will be the ability to identify new surrogate endpoints, such as persistently low vector copy numbers, which likely means there is insufficient healthy hemoglobin production to modify the disease course. Because there are many unique ongoing trials, a stopping rule would likely have to consider outcomes other than just safety and efficacy, she said. Finally, Kanter added, investigators will need to monitor gene therapy recipients over the long term to see if these therapies provide long-term disease management or a cure and to determine how to make this type of therapy available, affordable, and universal.

DISCUSSION

A moderated panel discussion and question period with the workshop audience followed the presentations. Topics explored during this panel included patient perspectives on clinical endpoints, endpoint validation, and the costs associated with endpoint research.

Leveraging Patient Perspectives and Data

"How do patients feel about the endpoints used in clinical trials for Pompe disease?" a workshop participant asked, noting that tests such as the 6-minute walk test are not very popular among patients with neuromuscular diseases. There are perhaps more clinically relevant endpoints available, Koeberl said, such as the gait, stairs, gower, chair assessment, which has been validated and also correlates to the 6-minute walk test, so it will likely be used in the future. Developing more disease-specific endpoints will also be important, he added.

When asked to comment on why she thinks there is no national registry for sickle cell disease patients, Kanter replied that it comes down to decentralized patient advocacy for this condition and a lack of funding. She said that there are several groups starting to put together different forms of a registry, so collaboration is going to be key. "We want to make sure that too many people are not in the kitchen cooking up different registries," she said. In recent years the American Society of Hematology has undertaken sickle cell disease as its first disease-specific initiative, which is making a difference, she said, as has NIH and NHLBI's embrace of this disease, although the institutes have indicated they are not interested in being the long-term funder of a registry.

Developing and Validating Endpoints for Gene Therapies

Will there be a time, a workshop participant asked, when the resolution of anemia in sickle cell disease will become an accepted endpoint, just as the resolution of hypertension is the endpoint for drugs designed to lower blood pressure instead of a reduction in the incidence of stroke? It will be important, Lapteva answered, to demonstrate how improving anemia correlates with reduced disease burden, such as by reducing hospitalization, improving respiratory function, and reducing fatigue. "There are all of these ways to look at the reduction of the disease burden from the perspective of how you improve the symptoms," she added. "If you start thinking about it from that perspective, then there are ways to potentially look and validate the endpoint that you are talking about in terms of how it improves the outcomes in a patient." Kanter said that it can take years for those downstream patient outcomes to improve, which raises concerns in the sickle cell disease community that the validation of a surrogate endpoint, such as normal hemoglobin production, will take a very long time.

One participant asked how companies can get regulatory feedback on novel outcome measures outside of a development program. Lapteva answered that FDA has programs called the Drug Development Tool Qualification Programs,[7] which are meant to assess measures in a pre-competitive environment when there is no worry about disclosing proprietary information.

A participant asked whether microperimetry, which has the ability to interrogate the same point on the retina over time and has high sensitivity to variable light levels, might have the potential to serve as a sensitive measure of retinal disease over time. Many groups are working to validate measures like pupillometry as a surrogate endpoint, Maguire answered, but doing so will require correlating measurements with patient functional activity, such as an improved ability to walk around town.

Panelists were asked for their opinion of the statement that it is not possible to validate a surrogate endpoint in a rare disease. With many rare diseases, Maguire said, the timeline is so long that it is difficult for patients

---

[7]Additional information is available at https://www.fda.gov/drugs/development-approval-process-drugs/drug-development-tool-qualification-programs (accessed December 12, 2019).

and researchers alike to stay engaged and to find funding sources that are willing to commit to long-term studies that might last 5 or 10 years. The larger number of sickle cell disease patients makes it possible to validate surrogate endpoints for that disease, Kanter said, but the biggest obstacle is the lack of a national registry. "We would have a much better understanding of what in a 2-year-old would predict mortality in a 25-year-old if we had a longitudinal registry," she said. Koeberl added that there may be a couple of good surrogate endpoint candidates for retinal diseases, and it is just a matter of time to collect the data and confirm validation.

Endpoints are critical, a workshop participant said, but the costs of endpoint research will be significant. How is the field thinking about this? Maguire said that young investigators will likely not choose the topic because of the issues with funding. Maintaining a long-term focus and encouraging researchers and funders to consider endpoint development and research is challenging, he added. Sickle cell disease is somewhat different in that endpoints are a popular topic, Kanter said. In academia and in various organizations, the importance of endpoints needs to be realized in order to continue this type of research, she said. And High added, "I think we should really not underestimate the challenges involved in coming up with new endpoints that are really accepted by the clinical community, by regulators, and so forth." This is a crucial piece of developing gene therapies, she said.

5

Integrating Gene-Based Therapies into Clinical Practice: Exploring Long-Term Clinical Follow-Up of Patients

---

Important Points Highlighted by Individual Speakers

- The Food and Drug Administration (FDA) may require long-term follow-up for gene therapy products because they are intended to achieve a prolonged or permanent therapeutic effect and, as such, long-term exposure may produce unpredictable or unexpected delayed risks for a patient receiving that therapy. (Purohit-Sheth)
- Products that FDA considers to have a greater risk of delayed adverse events include those that use integrating viruses, viruses capable of latency reactivation, and genome-editing products. Products that FDA considers as having a lower risk of delayed adverse events include those using plasmids, poxvirus, adenovirus, and adeno-associated viruses because these approaches (while modifying expression of genes) do not produce lasting changes to the genome. (Purohit-Sheth)
- Informed consent should explain the purpose of the long-term follow-up study, the expected participation and procedures, foreseeable risks, scheduled study visits, and tissue and data collection procedures as well as the basic elements required for any clinical study. (Purohit-Sheth)
- Various mobile health applications combined with machine learning and artificial intelligence may also provide long-term insights into the health and outcomes of patients who take part

---

in gene therapy clinical trials. Mobile health applications may also encourage higher participation rates and more frequent reporting of symptoms by patients. (Robison)

- In terms of educating patients and motivating them to remain engaged during long-term follow-up, it would be helpful to enlist patients in a care program once they complete a clinical trial and to give them a summary of all of their treatments. (Robison)
- Regulatory agencies need to provide more clarity on the best methods for monitoring for off-target effects of genome editing and insertional mutagenesis. (Chonzi)
- Finding ways to combine long-term follow-up data with data from the post-marketing experience would be helpful for sponsors and allow for the harmonization of data collection methods and approaches to following patients. (Chonzi)
- Patient groups with strong infrastructure and registries can help facilitate a robust post-marketing research program. The Cystic Fibrosis Foundation has been successful in this area in large part due to strong business relationships with pharmaceutical sponsors and credibility with regulatory agencies with regard to the patient registry. (Marshall)

The workshop's next session explored the implications of the long-term clinical management of patients who participate in gene-based clinical trials and discussed how data from a limited number of patients can be used effectively to determine if a gene-based therapy is safe and effective. The session was moderated by Michael DeBaun, a professor of pediatrics and medicine, the vice chair for clinical and translational research, and the J.C. Peterson Endowed Chair in Pediatric Pulmonology at Vanderbilt University and director of the Vanderbilt-Meharry Center for Excellence in Sickle Cell Disease. Tejashri Purohit-Sheth, the director of the Division of Clinical Evaluation, Pharmacology, and Toxicology in the Office of Tissues and Advanced Therapies, Center for Biologics Evaluation and Research at FDA, discussed the agency's recommendations regarding long-term follow-up of gene-based therapies. Leslie Robison, the chair of the Department of Epidemiology and Cancer Control and a co-leader of the Cancer Control and Survivorship Program at St. Jude Children's Research Hospital, spoke about his experience with the long-term surveillance of pediatric and adolescent cancer survivors. David Chonzi, the vice president for pharmacovigilance and epidemiology at Allogene, addressed long-term follow-up for gene and cellular therapies. Bruce Marshall, the senior vice president of clinical affairs at the Cystic Fibrosis Foundation, discussed the foundation's role in addressing post-approval regulatory obligations. Bob Levis, one of the early recipients of experimental chimeric antigen receptor T cell (CAR T) therapy for chronic lymphocytic leukemia (CLL), provided a patient's perspective on long-term follow-up studies.

PERSPECTIVES FROM THE FOOD AND DRUG ADMINISTRATION ON LONG-TERM FOLLOW-UP STUDIES

In her presentation, Purohit-Sheth summarized FDA's July 2018 draft guidance, *Long-Term Follow-Up After Administration of Human Gene Therapy Products*.[1] Long-term follow-up, she explained, refers to monitoring for adverse events for an extended period of time, which is specified in the clinical studies protocol. The follow-up is meant for individuals who were in clinical studies following the completion of the study as well as for patients receiving gene therapy products after FDA approval. Depending on the risk characteristics of a specific product and what the agency understands about that product, it may not require long-term follow-up, she added.

FDA may require long-term follow-up for gene therapy products because they are intended to achieve a prolonged or permanent therapeutic effect and, as such, long-term exposure may produce unpredictable or unexpected delayed risks for a patient receiving that therapy. Delayed risks can include malignancy, impaired gene function, autoimmune-like reactions, a reactivation after latency and infection, and resistant infections. All of these potential delayed risks depend on the type of vector used in the gene therapy product, Purohit-Sheth said. FDA takes the following characteristics into account when determining which gene therapy products have an increased risk for adverse events:

- the integration activity of the product,
- whether it is a gene-editing construct,
- if the transgene is expressed for a prolonged time,
- if the potential for latency exists, such as with replication-competent herpes virus vectors, and
- if the vector establishes a persistent infection, as occurs with listeria vectors.

---

[1]The draft guidance is available at https://www.fda.gov/regulatory-information/search-fda-guidance-documents/long-term-follow-after-administration-human-gene-therapy-products (accessed December 23, 2019).

In general, Purohit-Sheth said, the products that FDA considers to have a greater risk of delayed adverse events include those that use integrating viruses, viruses capable of latency reactivation, and genome-editing products. Products considered to have a lower risk of delayed adverse events include those using plasmids, poxvirus, adenovirus, and AAVs. However, if a plasmid has been modified to have the ability to transfer or modify genetic elements, it may be considered to be a higher-risk product, she said.

As part of its draft guidance, FDA has developed a framework to assess the risk of delayed adverse events associated with a gene therapy product (see Figure 5-1). As part of its risk assessment, FDA looks at preclinical data to provide information about the localization, distribution, and persistence of the gene therapy product and to understand possible on-target and off-target effects. When designing preclinical studies, it is important to take into account the gene therapy formulation and the route of administration intended for human use, Purohit-Sheth said. Such studies should also evaluate the product in both male and female animals and evaluate whether product persistence and localization correlate with any adverse effects that may have been muted. Biodistribution studies should use the maximum feasible or clinical dose, and preclinical work should also include kinetic studies. FDA recommends that animal sacrifice should occur at the peak of

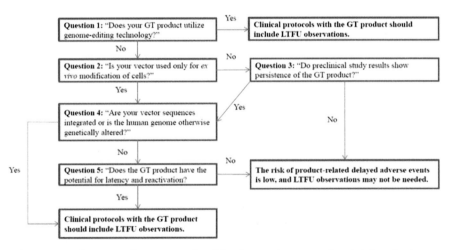

FIGURE 5-1 Framework to assess the risk of gene therapy–related delayed adverse events.
NOTE: GT = gene therapy; LTFU = long-term follow-up.
SOURCES: Tejashri Purohit-Sheth workshop presentation, November 13, 2019. Originally from the FDA draft guidance document *Long-Term Follow-Up After Administration of Human Gene Therapy Products* (p. 6).

gene therapy product detection and at later timepoints to provide information on product clearance.

Preclinical studies should contain a minimum tissue panel analysis that includes blood and tissue from the injection sites, gonads, brain, liver, kidneys, lung, heart, and spleen as well as additional tissues dependent on the product, vector type and tropism, and the route of administration, Purohit-Sheth said. It is critical when assessing vector persistence and distribution that the assay methodology be both quantitative and sensitive, she said. Assays should be able to detect vector sequences in both animals and humans.

Turning to the subject of clinical considerations for long-term follow-up studies, Purohit-Sheth said that the agency considers the goals of long-term follow-up, choice of subjects, and study duration. Informed consent for trials that include long-term follow-up will have to include provisions for post-trial consent. The goals of long-term follow-up, she said, are to identify delayed risks associated with exposure to the gene therapy product and to gain insights into the persistence of the gene therapy in the body. The long-term follow-up population, she added, will include all subjects who received the gene therapy in a clinical trial. When designing the long-term follow-up protocol, it is important to consider life expectancy based on the underlying disease, the possibility of multiple comorbidities, and exposure to other agents such as radiation and chemotherapy, which can have their own long-term adverse effects. The duration of a follow-up study should be sufficient to assess any possible adverse events, taking into account the product's characteristics, such as the observed duration of in vivo product persistence, the observed duration of transgene expression, and other in vivo product characteristics observed during preclinical and clinical studies.

Other considerations include the nature of the exposure to the product, its target organ or cell, and expected survival rates and known background rates of survival in the study population. For integrating vectors and genome-editing products, FDA recommends that long-term follow-up studies should last for 15 years, while for AAV vectors, FDA recommends a 5-year follow-up period. All follow-up studies should proceed using a dedicated clinical protocol with prespecified patient visit schedules, a prespecified sampling plan, the methodology that will be used to assess the persistence of vector sequences, the clinical events that will be monitored, a means of collecting accurate case histories, and a health care provider template for non-investigator caregivers. The protocol should also specify how adverse events will be reported to FDA, how they will be discussed in annual reports, and the procedure for submitting any necessary protocol amendments, such as the need to assess a new risk.

For the first 5 years of a long-term follow-up study, FDA recommends having a detailed plan for scheduled visits and the information to be collected at each visit. Case histories, Purohit-Sheth said, should contain information about any exposure to mutagenic agents and the emergence of new medical conditions of interest. Over the subsequent 10 years, FDA recommends contacting subjects at least yearly by phone, office visit, or questionnaire.

Informed consent should explain the purpose of the long-term follow-up study, the expected participation and procedures, foreseeable risks, scheduled study visits, and tissue and data collection procedures as well as the basic elements required for any clinical study. It is important to explain the possible adverse events so that the patient can understand the risks and know what to look for over time, Purohit-Sheth said. Informed consent should also include a request, in the event of a patient's death, for consent for autopsy. On a final note, she said that FDA discusses with applicants at the time they submit their biologics licensure application that they will need to have a post-marketing pharmacovigilance plan that includes routine surveillance. Depending on a particular product's risks, a risk evaluation and mitigation strategy may also be required.

LONG-TERM SURVEILLANCE OF EXPOSED PEDIATRIC AND ADOLESCENT CANCER SURVIVORS

Survival rates for childhood cancer in the United States are exceptional, Robison said, with 5-year survival rates now exceeding 83 percent. Approximately 1 in 750 U.S. residents is a childhood cancer survivor, with the number of survivors expected to approach 500,000 by 2020 (Robison and Hudson, 2014). Robison noted that this is a small, heterogeneous population for which there are recognized long-term consequences related to the treatment these individuals received as children. To better understand those consequences, the National Cancer Institute (NCI) has funded two large childhood cancer cohorts: the Childhood Cancer Survivor Study (CCSS) cohort of nearly 36,000 survivors from 31 centers across the United States and the St. Jude Lifetime (SJLIFE) cohort of more than 8,200 survivors (see Table 5-1).

The CCSS cohort, now in its 24th year, was originally assembled in response to the realization that many pediatric cancer survivors were not being actively surveilled, Robison said. The majority of the cohort participants had been involved in clinical trials through NCI's Cooperative Clinical Trials groups, but two-thirds of the patients who had been diagnosed and treated between 1970 and 1985 had not been seen by a pediatric oncologist for more than 10 years. CCSS is currently following more than 24,000 survivors who are distributed geographically across the nation, which Robison said creates some significant challenges in terms of monitoring, contacting, and overall follow-up. The SJLIFE cohort includes

TABLE 5-1 Pediatric Cancer Survivor Cohort Characteristics

Characteristic	CCSS (Dx 1970–1999)	SJLIFE (Dx 1962–2012)
Cohort size	35,937 (24,000+ active participants)	8,245 (4,688 participants to date)
Entry criteria	≥5 years from diagnosis	≥5 years from diagnosis
Age at cancer diagnosis	<21 years	<25 years
Cancers	Leukemia, CNS, HL, NHL, neuroblastoma, soft tissue sarcoma, Wilms, bone tumors	All diagnoses
Study design	Retrospective cohort with prospective follow-up, hospital-based	Retrospective cohort with prospective follow-up, hospital-based
Methods of contact	Surveys	Clinic visits and surveys
Comparison population	Siblings, general population	Frequency-matched community controls, general population
Therapeutic exposures	>90%	100%
Ascertainment methods	Self-report, pathology reports, NDI	Med. assessment, self-report, med. record, NDI
Collection of germline DNA	>60%	>95%

NOTE: CCSS = Childhood Cancer Survivor Study; CNS = central nervous system; Dx = diagnosis; HL = Hodgkin lymphoma; NDI = National Death Index; NHL = non-Hodgkin lymphoma; SJLIFE = St. Jude Lifetime.
SOURCE: Leslie Robison workshop presentation, November 13, 2019.

only patients diagnosed and treated at St. Jude Children's Research Hospital since the institution opened its doors in 1962. All of the participants in both cohorts are at least 5-year cancer survivors.

The CCSS cohort, Robison said, is completely survey-based, with most of the data self-reported by the participants. The SJLIFE cohort is clinically based, with participants returning to the hospital for 3 to 4 days of evaluation. Both cohorts have comparison populations to provide an idea of what events might be expected to occur normally over time and at what rate in an appropriate age-, sex-, and race-matched population. The CCSS cohort uses siblings as its control group, which Robison said is very good for evaluating certain aspects while not as good for evaluating psychosocial or sociodemographic outcomes. SJLIFE, on the other hand, relies on a community control group. For both cohorts, Robison and his colleagues collect detailed therapeutic exposure information and tissue samples that are banked for future study.

Addressing the challenges of assembling a cohort retrospectively, Robison said that 18 percent of the potential CCSS participants either never responded to attempts to reach them or actively refused to participate. Of the approximately 14,000 survivors who initially agreed to join the cohort, 1,300 provided extensive self-reported health information but declined to sign a medical release allowing the researchers to obtain their complete medical records. Ultimately, Robison said, only 72 percent of the eligible population was successfully recruited to join the study, a rate of success that he believes would have been higher had those individuals not been lost in the first place. "We are advocating very strongly that, going forward, this should be done on a prospective basis, consenting at the completion of therapy and starting to collect information on a periodic basis going forward," Robison said.

One of the strengths of assembling a cohort of survivors, Robison said, is that it is possible to look at multiple outcomes, which is important, given that pediatric cancer survivors are at risk for many different types of adverse outcomes. Data from the SJLIFE cohort revealed that the prevalence of a variety of adverse events, such as the occurrence of abnormal pulmonary function, hearing loss, heart valve disorder, and breast cancer in female survivors, increased over time and that, when assessed in the clinic, survivors were found to be experiencing multiple health issues (Bhakta et al., 2017). "By 45 years of age, on average, a survivor will experience approximately four severe, disabling, or life-threatening conditions," Robison said. For measuring long-term outcomes, he added, the control group is very important for understanding how much of an increased risk of morbidity there may be for pediatric cancer patients.

Bringing patients back to the clinic for follow-up studies would probably not have been realistic, Robison said, without the very large philanthropic support his team has received for studying the SJLIFE cohort. It is possible to link the cohort to the National Death Index to identify individuals who may be lost to follow-up, and NCI is in the process of creating a virtual national cancer registry that can be used to identify whether any cohort member is subsequently diagnosed with cancer anywhere in the United States. His team has also linked to organ transplant and assisted reproduction registries, but, he said, long-term follow-up in the United States is limited compared with other countries where there is high-quality record linkage.

Various mobile health applications combined with machine learning and artificial intelligence may also provide long-term insights. Robison's team, for example, is starting to rely on a mobile health application for self-reporting symptoms on a regular basis. This approach has enabled the team to achieve high participation rates for self-reporting of symptoms on a daily basis and of the symptoms' impact on quality of life on a monthly basis.

In closing, Robison said that his team is very interested in looking at the lifetime outcomes in order to better understand whether pediatric and adolescent cancer survivors, as a result of their cancer and treatment exposures, experience an earlier onset of disease and morbidity than the general population. Concerning gene therapy follow-up, he said that it will be important to have long-term and constant surveillance because there will likely be emerging and late-occurring events within those populations.

LONG-TERM FOLLOW-UP FOR GENE AND CELLULAR THERAPIES

Long-term follow-up for cellular therapies, Chonzi said, should include monitoring for adverse events such as secondary malignancies, autoimmune disorders, new persistent hematological disorders, and other issues such as hypogammaglobulinemia and infections. Following persistence is also important because it is not yet known if all cellular products have the same persistence characteristics in humans.

Before deciding whether to conduct a long-term follow-up study, Chonzi said it is important to ask several key questions:

- Does the product use genome-editing technology?
- Are vector sequences integrated, or is the human genome otherwise genetically altered?
- Does the product have the potential for latency and reactivation?
- Have any specific issues been raised during preclinical studies?
- How long will the study have to be run in order to detect the possible adverse events of interest and concern, particularly if secondary malignancies are a concern?

Because his organization is conducting studies globally, Chonzi said, it also has to pay attention to guidances issued by non-U.S. regulatory agencies. While those are largely consistent with FDA guidances, there are differences that create challenges for sponsors (e.g., guidance on replication-competent retrovirus testing after the first year).[2] "We are hoping that as time goes on there is going to be uniformity between the regulators as to how we monitor and follow our patients long-term," Chonzi said. Regarding CAR T therapy, most of the therapies use gamma retroviruses

---

[2]For more information, see the 2018 FDA guidance at https://www.fda.gov/regulatory-information/search-fda-guidance-documents/testing-retroviral-vector-based-human-gene-therapy-products-replication-competent-retrovirus-during (accessed January 24, 2020) and the 2009 European Medicines Agency guidance at https://www.ema.europa.eu/en/documents/scientific-guideline/guideline-follow-patients-administered-gene-therapy-medicinal-products_en.pdf (accessed January 24, 2020).

or lentiviruses to deliver CAR-encoding sequences into T cells, and these viruses can integrate or have the potential for latency followed by reactivation. Both CAR T products that are on the market have post-license, 15-year long-term follow-up studies ongoing, he noted.

Allogeneic CAR T therapies, which use genome-editing technology, are also under development and have entered clinical testing. At this point, Chonzi said, it is unclear if there will be differences in how autologous and allogeneic cellular therapies will be followed over the long term. Also unclear, he said, is how sponsors will follow integration and genotoxicity over the long term. It would be helpful if regulatory agencies provided more clarity on monitoring for the off-target effects of genome editing and insertional mutagenesis, Chonzi said. He also wondered if there is a way of combining long-term follow-up data from studies with data from the post-marketing experience. Doing so, he said, would allow for harmonizing the two collection methods and two approaches to following patients. Patients in studies could be enrolled in the same registries used for commercial purposes, Chonzi suggested, especially when patients finish the active follow-up of a study.

In closing, Chonzi emphasized the importance of having all stakeholders share their experiences and lessons from long-term follow-up studies. Some groups have done so, he said, but more data are needed on secondary malignancies, autoimmune disorders, and persistent hematological disorders. The field of cellular therapy is growing considerably, and more studies will be coming, he said, adding that "it is even more important for us at this moment in time to try and harmonize how we are collecting the data so that it becomes easier and easier."

ROLE OF THE CYSTIC FIBROSIS FOUNDATION IN ADDRESSING POST-APPROVAL REGULATORY OBLIGATIONS

Tracking patient outcomes after a gene therapy clinical trial may be improved through access to a patient registry. While there is currently no FDA-approved gene therapy for cystic fibrosis on the market, there are potentially important lessons to learn from the experience of the Cystic Fibrosis Foundation in building their patient registry and using it to follow clinical outcomes in the long term. The Cystic Fibrosis Foundation's patient registry, which was started in the 1960s, is one of the organization's crown jewels, Marshall told the workshop. Each night the 133 participating clinical centers download their data to the registry, which then provides analysis back to the centers through a Web-based application called CFSmartReports. The registry also allows for the generation of patient summary reports, population management reports, and clinical trial eligibility reports, all of which are helpful to clinicians because they bring registry data back to the point of care, Marshall said.

Another important way that the patient registry has been used is in supporting the pharmaceutical industry with post-marketing analyses, Marshall said. He added that FDA approvals of drugs to treat cystic fibrosis have come with post-approval requirements and commitments, which have included

- a 10-year prospective observational study to assess the risk of fibrosing colonopathy[3] for reformulated pancreatic enzymes;
- a 5-year prospective observational study to assess the risk of antibiotic resistance to a new inhaled antibiotic; and
- a 5-year prospective observational study to assess the safety of a new modulator of the cystic fibrosis transmembrane conductance regulator (CFTR).

For the first study, in which the goal was to determine the incidence of fibrosing colonopathy, one major challenge was getting all of the different sponsors to harmonize their protocols for identifying fibrosing colonopathy, Marshall said. Anonymized registry patients at participating sites served as the denominator in calculating the incidence rate, and those patients did not require separate consent, he said. The numerator was derived from an IRB-approved, patient-consented study in which suspected cases of fibrosing colonopathy were adjudicated by an expert review panel.

The inhaled antibiotic study, Marshall said, was also IRB-approved and patient consented. The sponsor of this trial established a central laboratory to collect annual respiratory cultures and a standardized approach to collecting and analyzing the specimens; the results of the trial were linked to clinical outcomes in the Cystic Fibrosis Foundation's registry. For this trial, FDA mandated testing for antibiotic susceptibility, but the sponsor and the Cystic Fibrosis Foundation both agreed it was also important to track clinical outcomes. The data collected in this study, which ended in 2019, did indicate that resistance patterns increased, but with no effect on clinical outcomes, Marshall said.

For the first CFTR modulator, which was approved in 2012, the sponsor conducted an observational study to evaluate the long-term safety of the product in patients with cystic fibrosis. This study used existing anonymized registry data to compare those on the drug to a propensity-matched com-

---

[3]Fibrosing colonopathy is a potential side effect of high doses of pancreatic enzymes (used to manage pancreatic insufficiency in cystic fibrosis patients) and is characterized by abdominal pain, vomiting, bloody or persistent diarrhea, and insufficient weight gain or weight loss (Atlas and Rosh, 2011).

parator group. The outcomes measured included lung function, pulmonary exacerbation and hospitalization rates, mortality, and the number of lung transplants. An interim analysis of the study data confirmed the effectiveness of this drug at reducing hospitalizations, pulmonary exacerbations, mortality, and the need for organ transplantation and for stabilizing lung function over time (Bessonova et al., 2018).

Looking to the future, Marshall said that over the next 5 years new CFTR modulators should increase the percentage of cystic fibrosis patients who benefit from therapy from about 6 percent to 91 percent. As these therapies are used in infants and life expectancy normalizes for cystic fibrosis patients, there will need to be new approaches to following these individuals over the long term, Marshall said.

In closing, Marshall credited the foundation's strong infrastructure, which has been in place since the 1960s, as a key factor for success in developing a registry that can facilitate a robust post-marketing research program. He also noted the importance of the ongoing relationships the foundation has with pharmaceutical sponsors. "They knew us. They knew of our Care Center Network, and they knew of our registry, so, it was easy to develop a business relationship with them," he said. "We also had credibility with the FDA in terms of our registry."

A PATIENT'S PERSPECTIVE ON LONG-TERM FOLLOW-UP STUDIES

As the fourth patient to receive CAR T therapy for CLL at Penn Medicine in 2013 and one of the first to receive a second round of CAR T therapy in 2017, Levis provided a patient's perspective of what it is like to participate in a clinical trial—and as he put it, be genetically modified.

First diagnosed with CLL in 2002, Levis was treated initially with the then-standard chemotherapy regimen, which kept his disease in remission for more than 3 years. When he relapsed to a very aggressive form of the disease, he joined a clinical trial testing a promising new antibody-based drug, but he was randomized to the comparison drug, which did not work for him. With 3 to 4 pounds of tumor burden, his platelet and hemoglobin levels falling dangerously low, and little time left to live, Levis joined the first trial for CLL CAR T therapy at the University of Pennsylvania.

On March 12, 2013, he received an infusion of his genetically modified T cells and was told to prepare for challenges ahead. "Sure enough, 8 days later I developed these fevers, was hospitalized, heart rate elevated," Levis recalled. "It was horrible." Eight days later, the fevers broke, and the 30 palpable lymph nodes had returned to normal. His hemoglobin and platelet levels had started rising, and a bone marrow biopsy conducted 1 month later showed no trace of the disease. "It is like magic," Levis said. "You cannot believe it. You have got your life back."

Unfortunately, the disease returned 3.5 years later as a slowly progressing form that responded to antibody-based therapy. However, there was still disease present in his bone marrow, so Levis opted to enroll in a second clinical CAR T trial, this time using a humanized construct that the team at Penn Medicine wanted to try along with the antibody-based drug he was taking. Today, he has no tumor burden, the percentage of CLL cells in his marrow has dropped from 40 percent to less than 5 percent, and he feels good on low-dose antibody therapy.

Thinking about long-term follow-up, Levis said he hopes that by continuing to be an "experimental patient at Penn Medicine," researchers will be able to start answering questions around resistance mechanisms, the need for memory cells for long-term persistence, the role of booster doses sometime after the initial infusion, and reactivation of the protective cells. He closed by repeating something his oncologist told him, which was that this is not even the end of the beginning, and there are new approaches on the horizon.

DISCUSSION

The presentations in the session were followed by a moderated panel discussion, which served as an opportunity for workshop participants to ask questions of the speakers. The panel discussion explored the length of time patients are followed after a gene therapy clinical trial, motivating factors for participation in follow-up studies, and costs for tracking patients over several years.

Determining the Ideal Length for Follow-Up

A workshop participant asked Purohit-Sheth how FDA came up with 15 years as the length of long-term follow-up for gene-based therapies and if it would be possible with more study to identify those patients at the highest risk of developing long-term adverse events rather than following every patient for 15 years. There was a case of secondary malignancy that occurred 14 years after exposure, Purohit-Sheth explained, which is how the 15-year number came about. Regarding learning about long-term risks and delayed adverse events, she said that the field is not yet at a place—as it is with small-molecule drugs—where there are solid expectations as to how these gene-based therapies will work over the long term. "As we procure more information, gain additional understanding," she said, "certainly there is a possibility that these recommendations may be updated in the future based on our understanding and our experience with these products."

A key question involves understanding what level of elevated risk is acceptable, Robison said. Childhood cancer survivors, for example, can have up to a 20-fold increased risk of experiencing long-term adverse events associated with their treatments. What, he asked, is the level of risk that is important for a given population? Is a two-fold increased risk for a serious adverse outcome acceptable? Is it 50 percent increase? Is it five-fold? It will be important to determine what is considered significant and important to monitor, he said. The ultimate goal, he added, will be to understand which particular patients are at high risk because of their individual characteristics and their treatment exposure.

Participation and Payment Challenges Associated with Long-Term Follow-Up

A workshop participant asked Robison what he thought are some of the important steps to take to motivate patients and families to stay involved in long-term follow-up studies. Robison answered that his team uses a number of approaches, but the most important is to educate patients and families and provide feedback so that they understand the importance of continuing to participate over the long term. He noted that the National Academies have recommended that every cancer patient, once they complete treatment, should have a care program that includes a summary of all of their treatments, and he suggested that this field should consider doing the same thing in the name of educating patients and their families.

One concern of Robison's that had not been addressed, he continued, is how to pay for long-term follow-up studies. One possibility would be to identify risks, demonstrate that those risks are real and targeted to a specific population, and include that information in treatment guidelines. Once that occurs, he said, insurers will have a harder time justifying not covering the cost of long-term surveillance for those outcomes. DeBaun, the session moderator, noted that a large percentage of children and adults in the United States receive health insurance from the government through Medicare or Medicaid. The likelihood of an adult or child with sickle cell disease participating in long-term follow-up with a knowledgeable provider after receiving a curative therapy is less than 1 percent, he said. "Unless FDA acknowledges these non-funded mandates with strategies to follow this vulnerable patient population," DeBaun said, "it is unlikely that we are going to capture these data even a year to 2 years after curative therapy."

6

Reflections on the Workshop and Potential Opportunities for Next Steps

Celia Witten, the deputy director of the Center for Biologics Evaluation and Research at FDA, moderated a short panel session at the end of the day to discuss potential paths forward to support the clinical development of safe and effective gene-based therapies and to summarize the lessons learned and topics discussed through the day. The panelists were Ron Bartek, Mildred Cho, Richard Finkel, Pat Furlong, Katherine High, and Julie Kanter. Panelists were asked to consider ideas emerging from the workshop discussions and suggest specific changes that could improve the design of gene therapy clinical trials and the overall experience for participants and their families.

POSSIBLE NEXT STEPS FOR IMPROVING THE DESIGN OF GENE THERAPY CLINICAL TRIALS

When asked to identify the important points that emerged during the workshop, High emphasized the benefits of understanding the natural history of a disorder that is being treated with gene therapy, developing and validating novel endpoints, and improving the experience of patients who participate in clinical trials. The number of work streams and the expense required to mount a successful clinical trial for a gene therapy is staggering, she said, particularly for those diseases for which there are no existing therapies. However, the future is bright for the development of gene therapies for diseases where it is fairly straightforward to quantify outcomes, such as with hemophilia, thalassemia, and sickle cell disease, she said.

Possible Ways to Improve the Clinical Trial
Experience for Patients and Families

In terms of the next steps that product developers could take to improve the design of clinical trials for gene therapies, Furlong suggested standardizing the inclusion criteria for trials and the methodology and parameters for testing patients for immunity to the vector virus being used in the gene therapy. In the case of Duchenne muscular dystrophy (DMD), she said, there are three companies conducting gene therapy clinical trials, and each company has different methods for testing immunity to the vector virus. Patients would benefit from a clear explanation of the immunity testing parameters being used and the rationale for doing so, Furlong said. In the same vein, she suggested standardizing the sequence of outcome measures and data collection across trials for each disease. Doing so, she said, will require trial sponsors to work closely with FDA.

Efforts should also be made to maximize the potential therapeutic benefit of the first-in-human dose, Bartek said, given that most gene therapies will involve a one-time treatment. Furthermore, he said, developers and regulators should maximize inclusiveness from the start of clinical research and include both adults and children in early research. This would require shifting the paradigm of demonstrating safety of a therapy in adults first, he said, but the treatment for certain conditions may be profoundly effective in younger patients.

Learning from the Past and Scaling Up

Another approach to improving gene therapy clinical trials, Cho said, involves developing the infrastructure needed to scale gene therapies so that they can be appropriately integrated into clinical practice. In the future there should be a focus on establishing a rationing strategy for these therapies, given that it will likely be necessary until full scale-up has been achieved. Another step forward, Cho said, will involve understanding why recent clinical trials with gene therapies have been successful whereas the previous 30 years of trials had little success. There are lessons to learn, she said, in terms of patient enrollment, setting endpoints, and patient selection. Also of importance, Cho said, is the fact that the institutions that conduct these trials, the researchers involved, and the trial sponsors may all have interests that may be either competing or aligned with the interests of patients and families in terms of enrollment, retention, and access to treatment. Finally, she said, it will be critical to address the disparities that exist in the way that trials are conducted and the social justice issues that result from those disparities, such as who is offered long-term follow-up care and why, a point that had been previously mentioned by DeBaun.

Patient, Family, and Physician Education

Improving education for patients and their families about trials, expectations, and risks is the most important change to make to improve the experience of participants in gene therapy clinical trials, Kanter said. More patients should be included in trials as evidence mounts that outcomes are good, she said, noting that she has more than 15 people on a wait list to participate in a trial at her center. Furlong agreed with the need for more education, noting that pediatric diseases are family diseases and that often children in trials are separated from their siblings and other relatives, who may have only a little understanding about what is happening. One way to address this is to bring the family into the clinic for at least one appointment with the patient to give family members a better sense of what their loved one is going through and to provide them with an opportunity to ask questions.

Physicians need additional education about gene therapies and related clinical trials too, High said. As investigational agents become products, she said, it can become apparent how limited the understanding of gene therapy is among some physicians. Finkel added that physician education needs to include ways to frame patient expectations for these treatments so as to avoid disappointment.

Ideas for Developing Clinical Endpoints in Different Ways

Panelists were asked by an audience member if they saw opportunities for groups to work together in the precompetitive space to develop new endpoints for gene-based therapy clinical trials. There is both the opportunity and the need to do this type of work, Finkel said, but the challenge will be getting support for this type of effort from sponsors. Often a therapy will enter the preclinical pipeline without validated reliable outcome measures in place, he said, and noted that patient advocates can play an important role in getting resources and support for developing outcome measures and conducting natural history studies. A workshop participant suggested that NCATS be involved in supporting pre-competitive efforts aimed at developing new endpoints for gene therapy trials. Another example of effective pre-competitive efforts, Lapteva said, involves the drug development tool (DDT) qualification programs at FDA.[1] The aim of this set of programs is to qualify DDTs and make them available in order to expedite drug development and regulatory applications.

---

[1] More information about FDA's Drug Development Tool Qualification Programs can be found at https://www.fda.gov/drugs/development-approval-process-drugs/drug-development-tool-ddt-qualification-programs (accessed January 27, 2020).

ONGOING CHALLENGES FOR
GENE THERAPY CLINICAL TRIALS

Each disease area is faced with the issue of identifying the optimal population to study, Finkel said, and, in fact, children may be the ideal first population to study in certain situations. There are also challenges with producing enough vector to treat patients on a dose per kilogram basis, which again would argue for starting trials in children, he said.

Jay Siegel, a former forum co-chair, added that another major challenge is that many of the diseases amenable to gene-based therapies are quite rare, which makes it difficult to secure the funding to develop and test a novel therapy. His hope is that as technology improves and as the field gains experience with successful vectors, development and manufacturing costs will fall.

FINAL REMARKS AND SUMMARY

Witten provided an overview of points highlighted by individual speakers throughout the workshop. The first session, she recalled, involved a robust discussion around natural history data and its uses, about dose selection, and the importance of transparency and careful assessment (see Box 6-1).

The second session explored issues of patient selection, enrollment, and consent both from the researchers' point of view and from the patients' perspective. The discussion, Witten said, focused on trial enrollment in the context of other available care, on burdens incurred by patients and their families during trial participation, and on eligibility criteria that can make trial enrollment difficult, Witten said (see Box 6-2).

The third session at the workshop included a robust discussion centered on developing endpoints for gene therapy clinical trials, Witten recalled. Examples were provided by speakers, including one that centered on developing a novel, clinically meaningful endpoint for assessing visual improvement in patients with retinal disorders. The workshop heard that patient registries can be valuable tools for developing clinical endpoints and that educational materials tailored to patients might be important to include in a given trial, Witten said. Additional points are provided in Box 6-3.

The fourth session of the workshop examined long-term patient followup and management. There is general agreement that long-term follow-up is needed in certain cases to identify and mitigate delayed risk, Witten said. Other fields, including oncology and cystic fibrosis, can provide excellent examples and lessons learned about challenges to following clinical trial participants and the transition from being a participant in a clinical trial to

---

BOX 6-1
Key Points from Individual Speakers Related to Natural History Data and First-in-Human Gene Therapy Clinical Trials

- Natural history data can be valuable for serving as a control and can inform the development of endpoints as well as the interpretation of safety and efficacy data. (Finkel, High, Kaufmann)
- Natural history datasets can be made more robust with frequent visits, standardized measures, and an effort to collect high-quality, patient-level data. (High, Kaufmann)
- When selecting a starting dose, consideration should be given to selecting a potentially effective dose. (Bartek, Finkel)
- When selecting the study population, it is important to identify the genetic diagnosis (if applicable) and to be aware of any effects on safety or efficacy with particular genotypes. (Finkel)
- Pediatric populations (infants, children, adolescents) are all different and exhibit differences in drug metabolism, excretion, presentation, and off-target effects, factors that are important when testing experimental gene therapies. (Finkel)
- Strong partnerships between patients, families, researchers, and clinicians are critical for collecting natural history data and moving the development of gene therapies forward. (Kaufmann)
- Trial design will need to take into account the unique aspects of each disease/condition, including what therapies are available, if any. (Finkel, Kimmelman)
- Although some early trials in small groups or a single patient may be performed with the aim of treatment, transparency and rigorous data collection are critically important in these cases as well. (Kimmelman)

---

surviving the disease and returning to standard clinical care, she said. The fourth session highlighted the need for strong infrastructure for long-term surveillance, Witten said, and there may be some exciting opportunities with mobile health applications. Summary points from the fourth session are provided in Box 6-4.

Over the years, the regulatory process has evolved with regard to gene therapies, Siegel said, and FDA is much more flexible regarding novel designs and approaches to clinical trials and the use of registries and surrogate endpoints, all while trying to maintain high scientific standards and make all of this feasible. The field is better situated today than at any time in the past to answer the challenges identified over the course of the day, he continued. "We know a lot more about how to create and develop registries and use them in the drug development and regulatory setting than we did," he said, "and we know a lot more about how to create endpoints and how to validate endpoints, whether surrogate or real endpoints."

BOX 6-2
Key Points from Individual Speakers Related to
Patient Selection, Enrollment, and Consent

- Patients and families should be team members or partners in the research and development process. (Furlong, Tisdale)
- The informed consent process for gene therapy trials can be confusing for patients and their families. A summary or abstract of the informed consent would be helpful, as would providing additional time for patients and families to ask questions of the researchers. (Fitzhugh, Furlong)
- Trust between patients, families, and those overseeing the clinical trials depends on open communication and must be developed over multiple interactions. (Samuels)
- Earlier treatment with gene therapies often results in better patient outcomes, and newborn screening can help identify infants with rare, serious conditions. (Bartek, Puck)
- Population-level newborn screening promotes fair access to treatment, including to cutting-edge trials. (Puck)
- Certain eligibility criteria, such as geography or age, and the lack of a sibling protocol can be restrictive or extremely challenging for patients and families. (Contreras, Furlong)
- Clinical trial participants and their families incur very high indirect financial costs. (Contreras, Furlong)
- Patients with sickle cell disease often must account for the potential burdens on their families of other treatment options in decisions about undergoing gene therapy trials. (Fitzhugh, Samuels)
- Many patients find value in having a support system available to them consisting of research nurses, physicians, and others who have gone through the trials. (Samuels)

BOX 6-3
Key Points from Individual Speakers Related to
Developing Endpoints for Gene Therapy Clinical Trials

- Clinically meaningful, reliable, and rigorous endpoints are especially important for gene therapy trials, where trials may be smaller and treatments are irreversible. (Lapteva, Maguire)
- Pompe disease and sickle cell disease are two examples of conditions that need improved clinical endpoints and predictors of disease severity. (Kanter, Koeberl)
- The multi-luminance mobility test provides a quantifiable and reproducible measure of clinically meaningful vision performance, but it was an expensive and lengthy investment to develop that measure. (Maguire)
- It is critical to define clinical trial "stopping points" for when a gene therapy is not working. (Kanter)
- Vector copy number and transduction levels can provide a predictive measurement of gene therapy. (Kanter)
- A collaborative, national sickle cell disease registry will be an important tool to help with development of reliable clinical endpoints. (Kanter)
- Educational materials for patients are critical to help convey that each gene therapy approach is unique with regard to the materials used, potential risks, and benefits. (Kanter)
- Investigators and sponsors working on rare disorders often find themselves defining novel endpoints midway through the development process. (Koeberl)
- Investigators or researchers who want a discussion with the Food and Drug Administration about the acceptability of their endpoint in a disease can consider participating in the agency's drug development tools program. (Lapteva)

BOX 6-4
**Key Points from Individual Speakers Related
to Long-Term Patient Follow-Up**

- Long-term follow-up is critical to identifying and mitigating delayed risks to patients who receive investigational gene therapies. (Purohit-Sheth)
- Retrospective follow-up presents several challenges, including the loss of contact with patients and patients' refusal to sign medical release documents; prospective approaches are preferable. (Robison)
- Mobile health applications may be useful tools to help with the collection of patient-reported outcomes over several years. (Robison)
- There is a need for further clarity on monitoring for the off-target effects of genome editing and insertional mutagenesis. (Chonzi)
- Harmonizing how long-term follow-up data are collected would help the field better understand potential risks. (Chonzi)
- Patient registries with a strong infrastructure are a valuable tool to help with post-marketing follow-up studies. (Marshall)
- Significant guidance on long-term follow-up is available from regulatory agencies around the world, including the Food and Drug Administration. (Chonzi, Purohit-Sheth)

References

Acland, G. M., G. D. Aguirre, J. Ray, Q. Zhang, T. S. Aleman, A. V. Cideciyan, S. E. Pearce-Kelling, V. Anand, Y. Zeng, A. M. Maguire, S. G. Jacobson, W. W. Hauswirth, and J. Bennett. 2001. Gene therapy restores vision in a canine model of childhood blindness. *Nature Genetics* 28(1):92–95.

Aslam, H. M., S. Yousuf, A. Kassim, S. M. Iqbal, and S. K. Hashmi. 2018. Hematopoietic stem cell transplantation for adult sickle cell disease in the era of universal donor availability. *Bone Marrow Transplant* 53(11):1390–1400.

Atlas, A. B., and J. R. Rosh. 2011. 81–Cystic fibrosis and congenital anomalies of the exocrine pancreas. In *Pediatric Gastrointestinal and Liver Disease* (4th edition). Philiadelphia, PA: Elsevier. Pp. 890–904.

Bennicelli, J., J. F. Wright, A. Komaromy, J. B. Jacobs, B. Hauck, O. Zelenaia, F. Mingozzi, D. Hui, D. Chung, T. S. Rex, Z. Wei, G. Qu, S. Zhou, C. Zeiss, V. R. Arruda, G. M. Acland, L. F. Dell'Osso, K. A. High, A. M. Maguire, and J. Bennett. 2008. Reversal of blindness in animal models of Leber congenital amaurosis using optimized AAV2-mediated gene transfer. *Molecular Therapy* 16(3):458–465.

Bessonova, L., N. Volkova, M. Higgins, L. Bengtsson, S. Tian, C. Simard, M. W. Konstan, G. S. Sawicki, A. Sewall, S. Nyangoma, A. Elbert, B. C. Marshall, and D. Bilton. 2018. Data from the U.S. and UK cystic fibrosis registries support disease modification by CFTR modulation with ivacaftor. *Thorax* 73(8):731–740.

Bhakta, N., Q. Liu, K. K. Ness, M. Baassiri, H. Eissa, F. Yeo, W. Chemaitilly, M. J. Ehrhardt, J. Bass, M. W. Bishop, K. Shelton, L. Lu, S. Huang, Z. Li, E. Caron, J. Lanctot, C. Howell, T. Folse, V. Joshi, D. M. Green, D. A. Mulrooney, G. T. Armstrong, K. R. Krull, T. M. Brinkman, R. B. Khan, D. K. Srivastava, M. M. Hudson, Y. Yasui, and L. L. Robison. 2017. The cumulative burden of surviving childhood cancer: An initial report from the St. Jude Lifetime Cohort Study (SJLIFE). *Lancet (London, England)* 390(10112):2569–2582.

Bond, J. E., P. S. Kishani, and D. D. Koeberl. 2019. Immunomodulatory, liver depot gene therapy for Pompe disease. *Cell Immunology* 342:103737.

Chan, Y. B., I. Miguel-Aliaga, C. Franks, N. Thomas, B. Trülzsch, D. B. Sattelle, K. E. Davies, and M. van den Heuvel. 2003. Neuromuscular defects in a Drosophila survival motor neuron gene mutant. *Human Molecular Genetics* 12(12):1367–1376.

Chung, D. C., S. McCague, Z.-F. Yu, S. Thill, J. DiStefano-Pappas, J. Bennett, D. Cross, K. Marshall, J. Wellman, and K. A. High. 2018. Novel mobility test to assess functional vision in patients with inherited retinal dystrophies. *Clinical & Experimental Ophthalmology* 46(3):247–259.

Chung, D. C., M. Bertelsen, B. Lorenz, M. E. Pennesi, B. P. Leroy, C. P. Hamel, E. Pierce, J. Sallum, M. Larsen, K. Stieger, M. Preising, R. Weleber, P. Yang, E. Place, E. Liu, G. Schaefer, J. DiStefano-Pappas, O. U. Elci, S. McCague, J. A. Wellman, K. A. High, and K. Z. Reape. 2019. The natural history of inherited retinal dystrophy due to biallelic mutations in the *RPE65* gene. *American Journal of Ophthalmology* 199:58–70.

Darras, B. T., T. O. Crawford, R. S. Finkel, E. Mercuri, D. C. De Vivo, M. Oskoui, E. F. Tizzano, M. M. Ryan, F. Muntoni, G. Zhao, J. Staropoli, A. McCampbell, M. Petrillo, C. Stebbins, S. Fradette, W. Farwell, and C. J. Sumner. 2019. Neurofilament as a potential biomarker for spinal muscular atrophy. *Annals of Clinical and Translational Neurology* 6(5):932–944.

De Sanctis, R., G. Coratti, A. Pasternak, J. Montes, M. Pane, E. S. Mazzone, S. D. Young, R. Salazar, J. Quigley, M. C. Pera, L. Antonaci, L. Lapenta, A. M. Glanzman, D. Tiziano, F. Muntoni, B. T. Darras, D. C. De Vivo, R. Finkel, and E. Mercuri. 2016. Developmental milestones in Type I spinal muscular atrophy. *Neuromuscular Disorders* 26(11):754–759.

Duque, S. I., W. D. Arnold, P. Odermatt, X. Li, P. N. Porensky, L. Schmelzer, K. Meyer, S. J. Kolb, D. Schümperli, B. K. Kaspar, and A. H. Burghes. 2015. A large animal model of spinal muscular atrophy and correction of phenotype. *Annals of Neurology* 77(3):399–414.

Feldkötter, M., V. Schwarzer, R. Wirth, T. F. Wienker, and B. Wirth. 2002. Quantitative analyses of SMN1 and SMN2 based on real-time lightcycler PCR: Fast and highly reliable carrier testing and prediction of severity of spinal muscular atrophy. *American Journal of Human Genetics* 70(2):358–368.

Finkel, R. S., M. P. McDermott, P. Kaufmann, B. T. Darras, W. K. Chung, D. M. Sproule, P. B. Kang, A. R. Foley, M. L. Yang, W. B. Martens, M. Oskoui, A. M. Glanzman, J. Flickinger, J. Montes, S. Dunaway, J. O'Hagen, J. Quigley, S. Riley, M. Benton, P. A. Ryan, M. Montgomery, J. Marra, C. Gooch, and D. C. De Vivo. 2014. Observational study of spinal muscular atrophy Type I and implications for clinical trials. *Neurology* 83(9):810–817.

Fitzhugh, C. D., M. M. Hsieh, D. Allen, W. A. Coles, C. Seamon, M. Ring, X. Zhao, C. P. Minniti, G. P. Rodgers, A. N. Schechter, J. F. Tisdale, and J. G. Taylor, 6th. 2015. Hydroxyurea-increased fetal hemoglobin is associated with less organ damage and longer survival in adults with sickle cell anemia. *PLOS ONE* 10(11):e0141706.

Fitzhugh, C. D., S. Cordes, T. Taylor, W. Coles, K. Roskom, M. Link, M. M. Hsieh, and J. F. Tisdale. 2017a. At least 20% donor myeloid chimerism is necessary to reverse the sickle phenotype after allogeneic HSCT. *Blood* 130(17):1946–1948.

Fitzhugh, C. D., M. M. Hsieh, T. Taylor, W. Coles, K. Roskom, D. Wilson, E. Wright, N. Jeffries, C. J. Gamper, J. Powell, L. Luznik, and J. F. Tisdale. 2017b. Cyclophosphamide improves engraftment in patients with SCD and severe organ damage who undergo haploidentical PBSCT. *Blood Advances* 1(11):652–661.

Foust, K. D., E. Nurre, C. L. Montgomery, A. Hernandez, C. M. Chan, and B. K. Kaspar. 2009. Intravascular AAV9 preferentially targets neonatal neurons and adult astrocytes. *Nature Biotechnology* 27(1):59–65.

Fung, M., Y. Yuan, H. Atkins, Q. Shi, and T. Bubela. 2017. Responsible translation of stem cell research: An assessment of clinical trial registration and publications. *Stem Cell Reports* 8(5):1190–1201.

Gao, Q. Q., and E. M. McNally. 2015. The dystrophin complex: Structure, function, and implications for therapy. *Comprehensive Physiology* 5(3):1223–1239.

Gluckman, E., B. Cappelli, F. Bernaudin, M. Labopin, F. Volt, J. Carreras, B. Pinto Simões, A. Ferster, S. Dupont, J. de la Fuente, J.-H. Dalle, M. Zecca, M. C. Walters, L. Krishnamurti, M. Bhatia, K. Leung, G. Yanik, J. Kurtzberg, N. Dhedin, M. Kuentz, G. Michel, J. Apperley, P. Lutz, B. Neven, Y. Bertrand, J. P. Vannier, M. Ayas, M. Cavazzana, S. Matthes-Martin, V. Rocha, H. Elayoubi, C. Kenzey, P. Bader, F. Locatelli, A. Ruggeri, M. Eapen, Eurocord, the Pediatric Working Party of the European Society for Blood and Marrow Transplantation, and the Center for International Blood and Marrow Transplant Research. 2017. Sickle cell disease: An international survey of results of HLA-identical sibling hematopoietic stem cell transplantation. *Blood* 129(11):1548–1556.

Haddad, E., B. R. Logan, L. M. Griffith, R. H. Buckley, R. E. Parrott, S. E. Prockop, T. N. Small, J. Chaisson, C. C. Dvorak, M. Murnane, N. Kapoor, H. Abdel-Azim, I. C. Hanson, C. Martinez, J. J. H. Bleesing, S. Chandra, A. R. Smith, M. E. Cavanaugh, S. Jyonouchi, K. E. Sullivan, L. Burroughs, S. Skoda-Smith, A. E. Haight, A. G. Tumlin, T. C. Quigg, C. Taylor, B. J. Dávila Saldaña, M. D. Keller, C. M. Seroogy, K. B. Desantes, A. Petrovic, J. W. Leiding, D. C. Shyr, H. Decaluwe, P. Teira, A. P. Gillio, A. P. Knutsen, T. B. Moore, M. Kletzel, J. A. Craddock, V. Aquino, J. H. Davis, L. C. Yu, G. D. E. Cuvelier, J. J. Bednarski, F. D. Goldman, E. M. Kang, E. Shereck, M. H. Porteus, J. A. Connelly, T. A. Fleisher, H. L. Malech, W. T. Shearer, P. Szabolcs, M. S. Thakar, M. T. Vander Lugt, J. Heimall, Z. Yin, M. A. Pulsipher, S.-Y. Pai, D. B. Kohn, J. M. Puck, M. J. Cowan, R. J. O'Reilly, and L. D. Notarangelo. 2018. SCID genotype and 6-month post-transplant CD4 count predict survival and immune recovery. *Blood* 132(17):1737–1749.

Han, S.-O., G. Ronzitti, B. Arnson, C. Leborgne, S. Li, F. Mingozzi, and D. Koeberl. 2017. Low-dose liver-targeted gene therapy for Pompe disease enhances therapeutic efficacy of ERT via immune tolerance induction. *Molecular Therapy—Methods & Clinical Development* 4:126–136.

Han, S.-O., G. Ronzitti, B. Arnson, C. Leborgne, S. Li, F. Mingozzi, and D. Koeberl. 2019. Erratum: Low-dose liver-targeted gene therapy for Pompe disease enhances therapeutic efficacy of ERT via immune tolerance induction. *Molecular Therapy—Methods & Clinical Development* 13:431.

Harlaar, L., J. Hogrel, B. Perniconi, M. E. Kruijshaar, D. Rizopoulos, N. Taouagh, A. Canal, E. Brusse, P. A. van Doorn, A. T. van der Ploeg, P. Laforêt, and N. A. M. E. van der Beek. 2019. Large variation in effects during 10 years of enzyme therapy in adults with Pompe disease. *Neurology* 93(19):e1756–e1767.

Hassell, K. L. 2010. Population estimates of sickle cell disease in the U.S. *American Journal of Preventive Medicine* 38(4 Suppl):S512–S521.

Holladay, J. T. 1997. Proper method for calculating average visual acuity. *Journal of Refractive Surgery* 13(4):388–391.

Hollister, B. M., M. C. Gatter, K. E. Abdallah, A. J. Armsby, A. J. Buscetta, Y. J. J. Byeon, K. E. Cooper, S. Desine, A. Persaud, K. E. Ormond, and V. L. Bonham. 2019. Perspectives of sickle cell disease stakeholders on heritable genome editing. *The CRISPR Journal* 2(6):441–449.

Janssen Pharmaceutica. 2020. *Addressing the challenges of drug discovery*. https://www.janssen.com/emea/drug-discovery (accessed January 12, 2020).

Koeberl, D. D., L. E. Case, E. C. Smith, C. Walters, S.-O. Han, Y. Li, W. Chen, C. P. Hornik, K. M. Huffman, W. E. Kraus, B. L. Thurberg, D. L. Corcoran, D. Bali, N. Bursac, and P. S. Kishnani. 2018. Correction of biochemical abnormalities and improved muscle function in a phase I/II clinical trial of clenbuterol in Pompe disease. *Molecular Therapy* 26(9):2304–2314.

Kolb, S. J., C. S. Coffey, J. W. Yankey, K. Krosschell, W. D. Arnold, S. B. Rutkove, K. J. Swoboda, S. P. Reyna, A. Sakonju, B. T. Darras, R. Shell, N. Kuntz, D. Castro, J. Parsons, A. M. Connolly, C. A. Chiriboga, C. McDonald, W. B. Burnette, K. Werner, M. Thangarajh, P. B. Shieh, E. Finanger, M. E. Cudkowicz, M. M. McGovern, D. E. McNeil, R. Finkel, S. T. Iannaccone, E. Kaye, A. Kingsley, S. R. Renusch, V. L. McGovern, X. Wang, P. G. Zaworski, T. W. Prior, A. H. M. Burghes, A. Bartlett, J. T. Kissel, and NeuroNEXT Clinical Trial Network on behalf of the NN101 SMA Biomarker Investigators. 2017. Natural history of infantile-onset spinal muscular atrophy. *Annals of Neurology* 82(6):883–891.

Lorson, C. L., H. Rindt, and M. Shababi. 2010. Spinal muscular atrophy: Mechanisms and therapeutic strategies. *Human Molecular Genetics* 19(R1):R111–R118.

Maguire, A. M., F. Simonelli, E. A. Pierce, E. N. Pugh, Jr., F. Mingozzi, J. Bennicelli, S. Banfi, K. A. Marshall, F. Testa, E. M. Surace, S. Rossi, A. Lyubarsky, V. R. Arruda, B. Konkle, E. Stone, J. Sun, J. Jacobs, L. Dell'Osso, R. Hertle, J.-X. Ma, T. M. Redmond, X. Zhu, B. Hauck, O. Zelenaia, K. S. Shindler, M. G. Maguire, J. F. Wright, N. J. Volpe, J. W. McDonnell, A. Auricchio, K. A. High, and J. Bennett. 2008. Safety and efficacy of gene transfer for Leber's congenital amaurosis. *New England Journal of Medicine* 358(21):2240–2248.

Maguire, A. M., K. A. High, A. Auricchio, J. F. Wright, E. A. Pierce, F. Testa, F. Mingozzi, J. L. Bennicelli, G.-S. Ying, S. Rossi, A. Fulton, K. A. Marshall, S. Banfi, D. C. Chung, J. I. W. Morgan, B. Hauck, O. Zelenaia, X. Zhu, L. Raffini, F. Coppieters, E. De Baere, K. S. Shindler, N. J. Volpe, E. M. Surace, C. Acerra, A. Lyubarsky, T. M. Redmond, E. Stone, J. Sun, J. W. McDonnell, B. P. Leroy, F. Simonelli, and J. Bennett. 2009. Age-dependent effects of *RPE65* gene therapy for Leber's congenital amaurosis: A phase 1 dose-escalation trial. *Lancet* 374(9701):1597–1605.

McWhorter, M. L., U. R. Monani, A. H. Burghes, and C. E. Beattie. 2003. Knockdown of the survival motor neuron (Smn) protein in zebrafish causes defects in motor axon outgrowth and pathfinding. *Journal of Cell Biology* 162(5):919–931.

MDA (Muscular Dystrophy Association). 2020. Duchenne Muscular Dystrophy (DMD). https://www.mda.org/disease/duchenne-muscular-dystrophy/causes-inheritance (accessed February 19, 2020).

Mendell, J. R., S. Al-Zaidy, R. Shell, W. D. Arnold, L. R. Rodino-Klapac, T. W. Prior, L. Lowes, L. Alfano, K. Berry, K. Church, J. T. Kissel, S. Nagendran, J. L'Italien, D. M. Sproule, C. Wells, J. A. Cardenas, M. D. Heitzer, A. Kaspar, S. Corcoran, L. Braun, S. Likhite, C. Miranda, K. Meyer, K. D. Foust, A. H. M. Burghes, and B. K. Kaspar. 2017. Single-dose gene-replacement therapy for spinal muscular atrophy. *New England Journal of Medicine* 377(18):1713–1722.

Mercuri, E., R. Finkel, J. Montes, E. S. Mazzone, M. P. Sormani, M. Main, D. Ramsey, A. Mayhew, A. M. Glanzman, S. Dunaway, R. Salazar, A. Pasternak, J. Quigley, M. Pane, M. C. Pera, M. Scoto, S. Messina, M. Sframeli, G. L. Vita, A. D'Amico, M. van den Hauwe, S. Sivo, N. Goemans, P. Kaufmann, B. T. Darras, E. Bertini, F. Muntoni, and D. C. De Vivo. 2016. Patterns of disease progression in type 2 and 3 SMA: Implications for clinical trials. *Neuromuscular Disorders* 26(2):126–131.

Monaco, A. P., R. L. Neve, C. Colletti-Feener, C. J. Bertelson, D. M. Kurnit, and L. M. Kunkel. 1986. Isolation of candidate cDNAs for portions of the Duchenne muscular dystrophy gene. *Nature* 323(6089):646–650.

Monani, U. R., M. Sendtner, D. D. Coovert, D. W. Parsons, C. Andreassi, T. T. Le, S. Jablonka, B. Schrank, W. Rossoll, T. W. Prior, G. E. Morris, and A. H. Burghes. 2000. The human centromeric survival motor neuron gene (SMN2) rescues embryonic lethality in SMN (-/-) mice and results in a mouse with spinal muscular atrophy. *Human Molecular Genetics* 9(3):333–339.

Naso, M. F., B. Tomkowicz, W. L. Perry, 3rd, and W. R. Strohl. 2017. Adeno-associated virus (AAV) as a vector for gene therapy. *BioDrugs: Clinical Immunotherapeutics, Biopharmaceuticals, and Gene Therapy* 31(4):317–334.

NIH (National Institutes of Health) Director's Blog. 2019. *A CRISPR approach to treating sickle cell.* https://directorsblog.nih.gov/2019/04/02/a-crispr-approach-to-treating-sickle-cell (accessed February 18, 2020).

NLM (National Library of Medicine). 2020. *What is gene therapy?* https://ghr.nlm.nih.gov/primer/therapy/genetherapy (accessed February 7, 2020).

Oskoui, M., G. Levy, C. J. Garland, J. M. Gray, J. O'Hagen, D. C. De Vivo, and P. Kaufmann. 2007. The changing natural history of spinal muscular atrophy type 1. *Neurology* 69(20):1931–1936.

Pai, S.-Y., B. R. Logan, L. M. Griffith, R. H. Buckley, R. E. Parrott, C. C. Dvorak, N. Kapoor, I. C. Hanson, A. H. Filipovich, S. Jyonouchi, K. E. Sullivan, T. N. Small, L. Burroughs, S. Skoda-Smith, A. E. Haight, A. Grizzle, M. A. Pulsipher, K. W. Chan, R. L. Fuleihan, E. Haddad, B. Loechelt, V. M. Aquino, A. Gillio, J. Davis, A. Knutsen, A. R. Smith, T. B. Moore, M. L. Schroeder, F. D. Goldman, J. A. Connelly, M. H. Porteus, Q. Xiang, W. T. Shearer, T. A. Fleisher, D. B. Kohn, J. M. Puck, L. D. Notarangelo, M. J. Cowan, and R. J. O'Reilly. 2014. Transplantation outcomes for sickle cell disease, 2000–2009. *New England Journal of Medicine* 371(5):434–446.

Paulukonis, S. T., J. R. Eckman, A. B. Snyder, W. Hagar, L. B. Feuchtbaum, M. Zhou, A. M. Grant, and M. M. Hulihan. 2016. Defining sickle cell disease mortality using a population-based surveillance system, 2004 through 2008. *Public Health Reports* 131(2):367–375.

Persaud, A., S. Desine, K. Blizinsky, and V. L. Bonham. 2019. A CRISPR focus on attitudes and beliefs toward somatic genome editing from stakeholders within the sickle cell disease community. *Genetics in Medicine* 21(8):1726–1734.

Quinn, C. T., Z. R. Rogers, T. L. McCavit, and G. R. Buchanan. 2010. Improved survival of children and adolescents with sickle cell disease. *Blood* 115(17):3447–3452.

Robison, L. L., and M. M. Hudson. 2014. Survivors of childhood and adolescent cancer: Lifelong risks and responsibilities. *Nature Reviews Cancer* 14(1):61–70.

Russell, S., J. Bennett, J. A. Wellman, D. C. Chung, Z.-F. Yu, A. Tillman, J. Wittes, J. Pappas, O. Elci, S. McCague, D. Cross, K. A. Marshall, J. Walshire, T. L. Kehoe, H. Reichert, M. Davis, L. Raffini, L. A. George, F. P. Hudson, L. Dingfield, X. Zhu, J. A. Haller, E. H. Sohn, V. B. Mahajan, W. Pfeifer, M. Weckmann, C. Johnson, D. Gewaily, A. Drack, E. Stone, K. Wachtel, F. Simonelli, B. P. Leroy, J. F. Wright, K. A. High, and A. M. Maguire. 2017. Efficacy and safety of voretigene neparvovec (AAV2-HRPE65v2) in patients with *RPE65*-mediated inherited retinal dystrophy: A randomised, controlled, open-label, phase 3 trial. *Lancet (London, England)* 390(10097):849–860.

Swoboda, K. J., T. W. Prior, C. B. Scott, T. P. McNaught, M. C. Wride, S. P. Reyna, and M. B. Bromberg. 2005. Natural history of denervation in SMA: Relation to age, SMN2 copy number, and function. *Annals of Neurology* 57(5):704–712.

Thein, S. L., and J. Howard. 2018. How I treat the older adult with sickle cell disease. *Blood* 132(17):1750–1760.

Thomas, C. E., A. Ehrhardt, and M. A. Kay. 2003. Progress and problems with the use of viral vectors for gene therapy. *Nature Reviews Genetics* 4(5):346–358.

Verhaart, I. E. C., A. Robertson, I. J. Wilson, A. Aartsma-Rus, S. Cameron, C. C. Jones, S. F. Cook, and H. Lochmüller. 2017. Prevalence, incidence and carrier frequency of 5q-linked spinal muscular atrophy—A literature review. *Orphanet Journal of Rare Diseases* 12(1):124.

Wang, R. T., F. Barthelemy, A. S. Martin, E. D. Douine, A. Eskin, A. Lucas, J. Lavigne, H. Peay, N. Khanlou, L. Sweeney, R. M. Cantor, M. C. Miceli, and S. F. Nelson. 2018. DMD genotype correlations from the Duchenne registry: Endogenous exon skipping is a factor in prolonged ambulation for individuals with a defined mutation subtype. *Human Mutation* 39(9):1193–1202.

Wendler, D., L. Belsky, K. M. Thompson, and E. J. Emanuel. 2005. Quantifying the federal minimal risk standard: Implications for pediatric research without a prospect of direct benefit. *JAMA* 294(7):826–832.

Xu, L., I. Irony, W. W. Bryan, and B. Dunn. 2017. Development of gene therapies-lessons from nusinersen. *Gene Therapy* 24(9):527–528.

Zarin, D. A., S. N. Goodman, and J. Kimmelman. 2019. Harms from uninformative clinical trials. *JAMA* 322(9):813–814.

Appendix A

Workshop Agenda

Exploring Novel Clinical Trial Designs for Gene-Based Therapies:
A Workshop

November 13, 2019

National Academy of Sciences Building
Lecture Room
2101 Constitution Avenue, NW
Washington, DC 20418

AGENDA

8:30 a.m.   **Opening Remarks**

KATHY TSOKAS, *Forum Co-Chair*
Regulatory Head of Regenerative Medicine &
    Advanced Therapy
Johnson & Johnson

8:35 a.m.   **Charge to Workshop Speakers and Participants**

KRISHANU SAHA, *Workshop Co-Chair*
Associate Professor
Retina Research Foundation Kathryn and Latimer
    Murfee Chair

Department of Biomedical Engineering
University of Wisconsin–Madison

8:45 a.m.   **Keynote Lecture**
Trial by "Firsts": Lessons from the Frontlines of
Clinical Trials in Gene Therapy

KATHERINE HIGH
President and Head of Research and Development
Spark Therapeutics

9:05 a.m.   **Clarifying Questions from Workshop Participants**

SESSION I: DEVELOPING FIRST-IN-HUMAN GENE THERAPY CLINICAL TRIALS

Session Objective:
- Explore the issues arising in the design of early-stage clinical gene therapy trials, including choice of endpoints, relevance, and requirements for preclinical data and identifying and using appropriate controls or natural history datasets.

Session Moderator: Cindy Dunbar, National Heart, Lung, and Blood Institute, National Institutes of Health

9:15 a.m.   JONATHAN KIMMELMAN
Director of Biomedical Ethics Unit
McGill University

9:30 a.m.   RICHARD FINKEL
Division Chief
Neurology
Department of Pediatrics
Nemours Children's Health System

9:45 a.m.   PETRA KAUFMANN
Vice President
R&D Translational Medicine
AveXis

10:00 a.m.   **Panel Discussion with Speakers and Workshop Participants**

10:30 a.m.   **Break**

SESSION II: UNDERSTANDING THE COMPLEXITIES OF PATIENT SELECTION, ENROLLMENT, AND THE CONSENT PROCESS

Session Objectives:
- Understand ethical issues surrounding patient selection, enrollment, and consent for gene-based therapies and how they differ from conventional clinical trials.
- Identify what resources are available to help patients and providers accurately understand the potential risks and benefits of participating in a gene-based clinical trial.
- Explore communication strategies aimed at helping patients make informed decisions about participating in trials for gene-based therapies.

Session Moderator: Mildred Cho, Stanford University

10:45 a.m.   COURTNEY FITZHUGH
Lasker Clinical Research Scholar
Laboratory of Early Sickle Mortality Prevention
National Heart, Lung, and Blood Institute
National Institutes of Health

11:00 a.m.   JOHN TISDALE
Senior Investigator and Director
Cellular and Molecular Therapeutics Laboratory
National Heart, Lung, and Blood Institute
National Institutes of Health

11:15 a.m.   JENNIFER PUCK
Professor, Department of Pediatrics
University of California, San Francisco

11:30 a.m.   PAT FURLONG
Founding President and Chief Executive Officer
Parent Project Muscular Dystrophy

11:45 a.m.   **Patient and Family Perspectives**
RON BARTEK

11:50 a.m.   MARÍA JOSÉ CONTRERAS

11:55 a.m.   TESHA SAMUELS

12:00 p.m.   **Panel Discussion with Speakers and Workshop Participants**

12:30 p.m.   **Working Lunch**

SESSION III: CONSIDERING THE CHALLENGES WITH DEVELOPING ENDPOINTS FOR GENE THERAPY CLINICAL TRIALS

Session Objective:
- Learn about successes and challenges in accurately measuring clinical endpoints and outcomes for gene-based therapies and moving products through the translational pathway.

Session Moderator: Larissa Lapteva, Food and Drug Administration

1:30 p.m.   LARISSA LAPTEVA
             Associate Director for Clinical and Nonclinical Regulation
             Division of Clinical Evaluation, Pharmacology,
                 and Toxicology
             Office of Tissues and Advanced Therapies
             Center for Biologics Evaluation and Research
             Food and Drug Administration

1:45 p.m.   DWIGHT KOEBERL
             Professor
             Department of Pediatrics/Division of Medical Genetics and
                 Department of Molecular Genetics and Metabolism
             Medical Director
             Biochemical Genetics Laboratory
             Duke University

2:00 p.m.   ALBERT MAGUIRE
             Professor of Ophthalmology
             Hospital of the University of Pennsylvania
             Presbyterian Medical Center of Philadelphia

2:15 p.m.   JULIE KANTER
             Associate Professor
             Hematology and Oncology
             University of Alabama at Birmingham School of Medicine

2:30 p.m.   **Panel Discussion with Speakers and Workshop Participants**

3:00 p.m.   **Break**

SESSION IV: INTEGRATING A GENE-BASED THERAPY INTO CLINICAL PRACTICE: EXPLORING LONG-TERM PATIENT MANAGEMENT AND FOLLOW-UP ISSUES

Session Objectives:
- Explore the implications of long-term clinical management of patients who participate in gene-based clinical trials (e.g., side effects, immunological implications).
- Discuss how data from a limited number of patients can be effectively used to determine if a gene-based therapy is safe and/or effective.

Session Moderator: Michael DeBaun, Vanderbilt University

3:15 p.m.   TEJASHRI PUROHIT-SHETH
Director
Division of Clinical Evaluation, Pharmacology,
    and Toxicology
Office of Tissues and Advanced Therapies
Center for Biologics Evaluation and Research
Food and Drug Administration

3:30 p.m.   LESLIE ROBISON
Chair
Department of Epidemiology and Cancer Control
Co-Leader
Cancer Control and Survivorship Program
St. Jude Children's Research Hospital

3:45 p.m.   DAVID CHONZI
Vice President
Pharmacovigilance and Epidemiology
Allogene

4:00 p.m.   BRUCE MARSHALL
Senior Vice President of Clinical Affairs
Cystic Fibrosis Foundation

4:15 p.m.   **Patient Perspective**
Bob Levis

4:20 p.m.   **Panel Discussion with Speakers and Workshop Participants**

SESSION V: NEXT STEPS AND WRAP-UP SESSION

Session Objectives:
- Discuss ways forward to support the clinical development of safe and effective gene-based therapies.
- Summarize the lessons learned and topics discussed throughout the workshop.

Session Moderator: Celia Witten, Food and Drug Administration

4:50 p.m.   **Final Panel Discussion**

Ron Bartek
Mildred Cho
Richard Finkel
Pat Furlong
Katherine High
Julie Kanter

5:20 p.m.   **Final Remarks from Workshop Co-Chairs**

CELIA WITTEN, *Workshop Co-Chair*
Deputy Director
Center for Biologics Evaluation and Research
Food and Drug Administration

5:30 p.m.   **Adjourn**
            Evening Reception – East Court

Appendix B

Speaker Biographical Sketches

Ronald Bartek, M.A., is the co-founder and the president of Friedreich's Ataxia Research Alliance, the chairman of the board of the National Organization for Rare Disorders, a 4-year member of the National Advisory Neurological Disorders and Stroke Council at the National Institutes of Health, and a former partner and president of a business and technology development, consulting, and government affairs firm. Mr. Bartek's professional experience also includes 20 years of federal executive branch and legislative branch service in defense, foreign policy, and intelligence, including 6 years on the policy staff of the House Armed Services Committee; 4 years at the Department of State's Bureau of Politico-Military Affairs, including 1 year as a negotiator on the U.S. Delegation to the Intermediate-Range Nuclear Forces Treaty talks in Geneva; 6 years as a Central Intelligence Agency analyst of political-military aspects of the East-West balance, including 1 year as an intelligence community representative to the interagency groups charged with U.S. arms control policy; and a former director of American Friends of the Czech Republic. Following graduation from the U.S. Military Academy at West Point, Mr. Bartek spent 4 years as an Army officer, serving as a company commander in Korea and an infantry and military intelligence officer in Vietnam. He has a master's degree in Russian area studies from Georgetown University.

Mildred Cho, Ph.D., is a professor in the Division of Medical Genetics of the Department of Pediatrics and in the Division of Primary Care and Population Health of the Department of Medicine at Stanford University. She is also the associate director of the Stanford Center for Biomedical

Ethics and the director of the Center for Integration of Research on Genetics and Ethics. She received her B.S. in biology in 1984 from the Massachusetts Institute of Technology and her Ph.D. in 1992 from the Stanford University Department of Pharmacology. Dr. Cho's major areas of interest are the ethical and social impacts of genetic research and its applications, including to precision medicine, gene therapy, the human microbiome, and synthetic biology. Her recent interests include the implications of applying data science, artificial intelligence, and mobile technologies to genomic and health data. She is a member of the Novel and Exceptional Technology and Research Advisory Committee of the National Institutes of Health.

David Chonzi, M.D., is the head of pharmacovigilance and epidemiology at Allogene Therapeutics, which is a clinical-stage biotechnology company pioneering the development of allogeneic chimeric antigen receptor T cell (CAR T) therapies for cancer. Prior to his role at Allogene Therapeutics, he was the global head of patient safety at Kite Pharma. He led the team that managed the safety profile for Yescarta, which is one of the first CAR T products to be approved by the Food and Drug Administration for treating advanced non-Hodgkin lymphoma. Dr. Chonzi spent 3 years at Roche-Genentech, where he led the patient safety team that was responsible for managing the safety profile for Tecentriq (anti-PDL-1) immune checkpoint. He holds an M.D. from the University of Zimbabwe as well as postgraduate qualifications in clinical pharmacology and epidemiology from the United Kingdom.

María José Contreras is from Chile. She is the mother of two boys affected by Duchenne muscular dystrophy: Franco (5 years old) and Julián (3 years old). In February 2019 she moved to the United States with her husband and sons to allow her son Franco to participate in a gene therapy clinical trial currently in development at Nationwide Children's Hospital in Columbus, Ohio.

Richard Finkel, M.D., is the chief of the Division of Neurology at Nemours Children's Hospital and a professor of neurology at the University of Central Florida College of Medicine in Orlando. He received his medical degree from the Washington University School of Medicine in St. Louis, Missouri, and completed his training in pediatrics, neurology, and neuromuscular medicine at Boston Children's Hospital and Harvard Medical School. Dr. Finkel held positions at the Children's Hospital Colorado and the Children's Hospital of Philadelphia before assuming his current position in Orlando in 2012. His clinical practice and research interests have focused on pediatric neuromuscular disorders, especially spinal muscular atrophy, Duchenne muscular dystrophy, inherited neuropathies, and neurometabolic disorders. Dr. Finkel has participated in numerous clinical trials, natural history studies, and the development of standard-of-care guidelines, and he has contributed to the development of outcome measures, clinical trial design, and biomarker identification for neuromuscular disorders. He has published more than 150 peer-reviewed manuscripts and book chapters. He is an associate editor of two neuromuscular journals and a co-editor of the current edition of *Swaiman's Pediatric Neurology* textbook. Dr. Finkel has been recognized for his contributions to translational research in spinal muscular atrophy by receiving the Bengt Hagberg memorial lectureship in 2017 and the Sidney Carter Award in Child Neurology from the American Academy of Neurology in 2018, and he shared the Zulch Prize from the Max Plank Institute in 2019.

Courtney Fitzhugh, M.D., received her B.S. magna cum laude from the University of California, Los Angeles, in 1996, and her M.D. from the University of California, San Francisco, in 2001. During medical school Dr. Fitzhugh participated in the National Institutes of Health (NIH) clinical research training program, where she studied with Dr. John Tisdale at the National Heart, Lung, and Blood Institute (NHLBI). After receiving her M.D., Dr. Fitzhugh completed a joint residency in internal medicine and pediatrics at the Duke University Medical Center, and in 2005 she did a combined adult hematology and pediatric hematology–oncology fellowship at NIH and Johns Hopkins Hospital. Dr. Fitzhugh returned to NHLBI in 2007 and was appointed as the assistant clinical investigator in 2012 and the clinical tenure track investigator in 2016. She is a member of the American Society of Hematology.

Pat Furlong is the founding president and the chief executive officer of Parent Project Muscular Dystrophy (PPMD), the largest nonprofit organization in the United States solely focused on Duchenne muscular dystrophy (DMD). Its mission is to end DMD. It accelerates research, raises its voice in Washington, demands optimal care for all young men, and educates the global community. DMD is the most common fatal genetic childhood disorder, and it affects approximately 1 out of every 3,500 boys each year worldwide. It currently has no cure. When doctors diagnosed her two sons, Christopher and Patrick, with DMD in 1984, Ms. Furlong did not accept "There's no hope and little help" as an answer. She immersed herself in DMD, working to understand the pathology of the disorder, the extent of research investment, and the mechanisms for optimal care. Her sons lost their battle with DMD in their teenage years, but she continues to fight—in their honor and for all families affected by DMD. In 1994 Ms. Furlong, together with other parents of young men with DMD, founded PPMD to change the course of DMD and, ultimately, to find a cure. Today, she continues to lead the organization and is considered one of the foremost authorities on DMD in the world.

Katherine High, M.D., is currently the president and the head of research and development at Spark Therapeutics, a biotech company that she co-founded in 2013. Under Dr. High's leadership, Spark received Food and Drug Administration approval of the first adeno-associated virus gene therapy product in the United States, a treatment for a rare form of congenital blindness. Dr. High was formerly a professor at the Perelman School of Medicine at the University of Pennsylvania, an investigator of the Howard Hughes Medical Institute, and the founding director of the Center for Cellular and Molecular Therapeutics at the Children's Hospital of Philadelphia. An elected member of the National Academy of Medicine and the American Academy of Arts & Sciences, she has published more than 200 scientific papers and holds a number of patents related to gene therapy.

Julie Kanter, M.D., is a lifespan hematologist specializing in sickle cell disease. Dr. Kanter is the director of the adult sickle cell disease program and the co-director of the comprehensive sickle cell research center at the University of Alabama at Birmingham. Dr. Kanter is very committed to improving outcomes in sickle cell disease and ensuring those outcomes reach the affected individuals. She works closely with national partners including the American Society of Hematology and the National Institutes of Health on both advocacy and research. Dr. Kanter works on the development of novel therapeutics in sickle cell disease with expertise in clinical trial recruitment and trial design as well as in areas of improving access to care.

Petra Kaufmann, M.D., is the vice president of research and development translational medicine at AveXis. Prior to joining AveXis, Dr. Kaufmann was the director of the National Center for Advancing Translational Sciences (NCATS) Office of Rare Diseases Research at the National Institutes of Health, where her work included overseeing the Rare Diseases Clinical Research Network program, the Genetic and Rare Diseases Information Center, and the Toolkit for Patient-Focused Therapy Development. Before joining NCATS, Dr. Kaufmann was the director of the Office of Clinical Research at the National Institute of Neurological Disorders and Stroke, where she worked with investigators to plan and execute a large portfolio of clinical research studies and trials in neurological disorders. This was where she also launched the Network for Excellence in Neuroscience Clinical Trials, a trial network to support scientifically sound, biomarker-informed phase 2 trials for neurological diseases in partnership with academia, industry, and patient groups. Dr. Kaufmann has spent most of her career at

Columbia University in New York City, where she trained in neurology and was a tenured faculty member. Her research focused on observational studies and trials in mitochondrial diseases and neuromuscular diseases including spinal muscular atrophy and amyotrophic lateral sclerosis. Dr. Kaufmann has served on the scientific advisory boards of numerous national and international organizations, and her research has resulted in more than 120 publications. A native of Germany, Dr. Kaufmann earned her M.D. from the University of Bonn and her master's degree in biostatistics from Columbia University's Mailman School of Public Health. Dr. Kaufmann is board certified in neurology and neuromuscular medicine.

Jonathan Kimmelman, Ph.D., is the James McGill Professor of Biomedical Ethics at McGill University and directs the biomedical ethics unit as well as his own research group, STREAM (Studies in Translation, Ethics and Medicine). Dr. Kimmelman's research centers on the ethical, policy, and scientific dimensions of clinical development. In addition to his book, *Gene Transfer and the Ethics of First-in-Human Experiments* (Cambridge Press, 2010), his major publications have appeared in *Science*, *JAMA*, *BMJ*, and *Hastings Center Report*. Dr. Kimmelman received the Maud Menten New Investigator Prize (2006), a Canadian Institutes of Health Research New Investigator Award (2008), and a Humboldt Bessel Award (2014), and he was elected a Hastings Center Fellow (2018). He has sat on various advisory bodies within the National Heart, Lung, and Blood Institute and the National Institute of Allergy and Infectious Diseases, served for four National Academies of Sciences, Engineering, and Medicine committees, and chaired the International Society of Stem Cell Research Guidelines for Stem Cell Research and Clinical Translation revision task force (2015–2016). His research has been covered in major media outlets, including NPR's *All Things Considered*, STATNews, and *Nature*. Dr. Kimmelman is the deputy editor at *Clinical Trials* and serves as an associate editor at *PLOS Biology*.

Dwight Koeberl, M.D., Ph.D., attended Carleton College and the Mayo Medical School and Graduate School and then moved to the University of California, San Francisco, for his pediatrics residency. He completed fellowship training in clinical and biochemical genetics at the University of Washington before joining the Division of Medical Genetics in the Department of Pediatrics at Duke University in 1999. He was recruited to Duke by Dr. Y.-T. Chen, who developed enzyme replacement therapy that became the standard of care for Pompe disease. He serves as the medical director for the Pediatrics Biochemical Genetics Laboratory and sees patients in the metabolic clinic. At Duke his research has focused on the development of new therapy for inherited metabolic disorders, especially for the glycogen storage diseases. He is currently developing drug and gene therapy for glycogen storage disease type I and type II; the latter is known as Pompe disease. In January 2019 he initiated a clinical trial of gene therapy for Pompe disease. His laboratory is developing gene editing with CRISPR for the glycogen storage diseases.

Larissa Lapteva, M.D., M.H.S., M.B.A., is the associate director in the Division of Clinical Evaluation, Pharmacology, and Toxicology in the Office of Tissues and Advanced Therapies of the Center for Biologics Evaluation and Research at the Food and Drug Administration (FDA). Since joining FDA in 2006, Dr. Lapteva has provided scientific and regulatory advice for clinical development programs with investigational new drugs, generic drugs, and biological products in various therapeutic areas, including products developed for the treatment of rare diseases. Dr. Lapteva is a practicing clinician and serves as faculty at the National Institute of Arthritis and Musculoskeletal and Skin Diseases at the National Institutes of Health, advancing the teaching mission of the institute for the next generation of physician-scientists. Dr. Lapteva received her degrees of master of health sciences from Duke University and master of business administration from the R.H. Smith School of Business.

Bob Levis, M.S., is a graduate of Grove City College (B.S., 1973) and the University of Illinois (M.S., 1975). His professional career includes 32 years with Air Products & Chemicals, Inc., including 22 years on overseas assignments in Brazil, Japan, Singapore, and Taiwan, where he was vice president and general manager of the company's largest division in Asia. Following retirement from Air Products, Mr. Levis also worked for ABEC (bioreactor manufacturer) as the director of business development in Asia, and he now consults for Asia & Brazil Connections, LLC. Mr. Levis was diagnosed with chronic lymphocyctic leukemia (CLL) while on his executive business assignment in Singapore in 2002. Following several years of treatments through remissions and relapses, his CLL became more aggressive. Without any other treatment options, he enrolled as one of the early experimental chimeric antigen receptor T cell (CAR T) patients in 2013 at Penn Medicine in Philadelphia. The first CAR T procedure put his CLL into complete remission for 3.5 years. He had a second CAR T while on ibrutinib at Penn Medicine in 2017, and his CLL is now a minimum residual disease and stable on ibrutinib. In addition to his board commitment to the CLL Society, Mr. Levis is on the Abramson Cancer Center Director's Leadership Council at Penn Medicine. He is also active with the biopharma industry and university research hospitals on patient advocacy initiatives and new CAR T science business development.

Albert Maguire, M.D., is a professor in the Department of Ophthalmology at the University of Pennsylvania Perelman School of Medicine, where he is a retina specialist and vitreo-retinal surgeon. He is also the attending physician for retina at the Children's Hospital of Philadelphia. Dr. Maguire is most well known for developing and carrying out the surgical procedures that are now used in a large number of gene therapy clinical trials testing interventions for blindness. He is also known for directing the first phase 1–3 gene therapy clinical trials for congenital blindness, which demonstrated efficacy and safety in children and adults. Dr. Maguire was instrumental in all of the proof-of-concept studies that first showed that gene-based intervention of blindness was possible. Results from the clinical trials that he directed led to the first approved gene therapy drug for genetic disease worldwide and the first Food and Drug Administration–approved recombinant virus-based gene therapy product for a genetic disease. Dr. Maguire's preclinical studies led to several gene therapy clinical trials other than the ones he directed. In the process he developed a gene therapy surgical training program that has certified retinal surgeons around the world for retinal gene therapy delivery. Dr. Maguire received a bachelor's degree in psychology from Princeton University and an M.D. from Harvard Medical School, and he completed an internship in surgery at the Yale University School of Medicine, a residency in ophthalmology at the Wilmer Eye Institute, Johns Hopkins University School of Medicine, and a combined medical/surgical fellowship in retina at William Beaumont Hospital, Royal Oak, Michigan. While serving as the chief resident at the Wilmer Eye Institute, he was recruited to the University of Pennsylvania and the Children's Hospital of Philadelphia. Dr. Maguire has received numerous awards, including the American Academy of Ophthalmology Achievement Award, the Paul Kayser International Award in Retina Research, the Association for Retinopathy of Prematurity and Related Diseases Award, the Retina Research Foundation Pyron Award, the Clinical Innovator Award (National Medical Association), and the Antonio Champalimaud Vision Award. Dr. Maguire has established a center for excellence in gene therapy at both the Children's Hospital of Philadelphia and the University of Pennsylvania Perelman School of Medicine, where patients with bi-allelic congenital blindness due to *RPE65* deficiency are now treated. He continues to run several other gene therapy clinical trials for blinding diseases. He is also co-director of the Center for Advanced Retinal and Ocular Therapeutics, a center that aims to develop treatments for a wide range of blinding diseases and to train the next generation of physician/scientists.

Bruce Marshall, M.D., is the senior vice president for clinical affairs at the Cystic Fibrosis Foundation. He joined the organization in 2002 and directs the clinically related activities of the foundation, including the care center network, quality improvement, clinical practice guidelines, the patient registry, and educational resources. Dr. Marshall was a tenured faculty member at the University of Utah School of Medicine, where he served as the founding director of the adult cystic fibrosis program from 1989 to 2002. Dr. Marshall earned a bachelor of arts degree at Johns Hopkins University and his medical degree at the University of Maryland School of Medicine. He earned a master's degree in medical management from Carnegie Mellon University.

Jennifer Puck, M.D., is a professor of immunology at University of California, San Francisco, where she cares for immunology patients and has a basic and translational research program focused on identifying genes and finding better treatments for severe combined immunodeficiency (SCID) and other rare human immune disorders. She has worked to develop newborn screening test for SCID, using T-cell receptor excision circles as a biomarker for T-cell development that can be measured in infant dried blood spots; this test has been adopted in all 50 states in the United States and in a growing number of countries. To study how outcomes can be improved for individuals affected with SCID and other single-gene immune disorders, Dr. Puck is the co-principal investigator of the Primary Immune Deficiency Treatment Consortium, a National Institutes of Health–funded network of 45 immunology and transplant centers in the United States and Canada. She is also working on clinical trials of lentivirus mediated gene therapy for X-linked SCID and Artemis-deficient SCID, the latter being a first-in-human trial.

Tejashri Purohit-Sheth, M.D., is currently the director of the Division of Clinical Evaluation and Pharmacology/Toxicology in the Office of Tissues and Advanced Therapies (OTAT) in the Center for Biologics Evaluation and Research at the Food and Drug Administration (FDA). She provides supervisory oversight for the clinical and pharmacology/toxicology review of submissions to OTAT. She previously served as the clinical deputy director in the Division of Anesthesiology, General Hospital, Respiratory, Infection Control and Dental Devices in the Office of Device Evaluation in the Center for Devices and Radiological Health at FDA as well as the acting division director and branch chief in the Office of Scientific Investigation in FDA's Center for Drug Evaluation and Research (CDER) and as a medical officer in the Division of Pulmonary, Allergy, and Critical Care at CDER. She completed an internal medicine residency at the Naval Medical Center Portsmouth, followed by a fellowship in allergy/immunology at the Walter Reed Army Medical Center. Following the fellowship, she took over as the service chief of the allergy/immunology clinic at the National Naval Medical Center in Bethesda, Maryland. Following her end of her obligated service as an active-duty naval officer, she transferred her commission to the U.S. Public Health Service and began her FDA career; currently she has served for 24 years as an active duty Uniformed Service officer.

Les Robison, Ph.D., received his Ph.D. in epidemiology from the University of Minnesota. He is currently the chair of the Department of Epidemiology and Cancer Control, the associate director of population sciences, and a co-leader of the Cancer Control and Survivorship Program within the Comprehensive Cancer Center at St. Jude Children's Research Hospital in Memphis, Tennessee. As a pediatric epidemiologist, Dr. Robison has had a career-long focus of etiologic and clinical research within pediatric populations, particularly childhood malignancies. He has conducted large national epidemiologic studies of childhood cancer and for 20 years was the founding principal investigator of the Childhood Cancer Survivor Study (a multi-institutional consortium evaluating a cohort of more than 40,000 5-year survivors of childhood cancer). Currently he is a co-principal investigator (with Dr. Melissa Hudson) of the St. Jude Lifetime Cohort Study (a clinical cohort of more than 8,000 survivors of childhood cancer treated at St. Jude). He holds current positions on numerous national committees, task forces, councils, and advisory boards in the fields of epidemiology, etiology, pediatric oncology, and cancer survivorship. Dr. Robison is the author of more than 700 original papers published in peer-reviewed journals.

Tesha Samuels is a patient who enrolled in Autologous Gene Therapy Transplant, a clinical trial at the National Institutes of Health (NIH), in 2017. Subsequently she received the transplant in March 2018. Since that time Ms. Samuels has returned to her full-time job with the District of Columbia city government, and because of the positive outcome with her clinical trial she dedicates part of her time to being an advocate for sickle cell research and clinical trial participation. Within the past year she has shared her story on several panels concerning sickle cell disease and clinical trials such as Rare Disease Day at NIH, the Howard University Cure Sickle Cell Symposium, and the Rare Disease Legislative Advocates congressional caucus briefing. Most recently she spoke to the House subcommittee on labor, health and human services, education, and related agencies.

John Tisdale, M.D., received his medical degree from the Medical University of South Carolina in Charleston after obtaining his B.A. in chemistry from the College of Charleston. He completed an internal medicine and chief residency at the Vanderbilt University Medical Center in Nashville and then trained in hematology in the Hematology Branch of the National Heart, Lung, and Blood Institute (NHLBI), where he served as a postdoctoral fellow. He joined the Molecular and Clinical Hematology Branch of NHLBI in 1998 and is now the chief of the Cellular and Molecular Therapeutics Branch. In 2011 the College of Charleston recognized Dr. Tisdale with the Alumni of the Year Award and the Pre-Medical Society's Outstanding Service Award in Medicine. He was recently elected to the American Society for Clinical Investigation and is a member of the American Society of Hematology. Dr. Tisdale's research and clinical work center on sickle cell disease. His group focuses on developing curative strategies for sickle cell disease through transplantation of allogeneic or genetically modified autologous bone marrow stem cells.

Appendix C

Statement of Task

Designing clinical trials to test the safety and efficacy of regenerative medicine therapies, such as gene- and gene-editing-based therapies, can be complex for several reasons, including challenges with determining an optimal dosage, delivering the product effectively, and successfully recruiting patients to what may be "single chance" trials, to name a few. To explore the design complexities and ethical issues associated with clinical trials for these types of therapies, an ad hoc planning committee will hold a 1-day public workshop in Washington, DC. Speakers at the workshop may be asked to discuss patient recruitment and selection for gene-based clinical trials, assessing the safety of new therapies, dose escalation, and ethical issues such as informed consent and the role of clinicians in recommending trials as options to their patients. The concept of repeat dosing and sensitization treatments may also be explored.

A broad array of stakeholders may take part in the workshop, including academic and industry researchers, regulatory officials, clinicians, bioethicists, and individuals/patients and patient advocacy groups. The planning committee will develop the workshop agenda, select and invite speakers and discussants, and may moderate the discussions. A proceedings of the workshop will be prepared by a designated rapporteur in accordance with institutional policy and procedures.

Appendix D

Registered Attendees

Sean Adler
Johns Hopkins University

Rachael Anatol
Food and Drug Administration

Eric Anthony
International Society for Stem
    Cell Research

Naomi Aronson
Blue Cross Blue Shield Association

Jane Atkinson
National Center for Advancing
    Translational Sciences

Dylan Bechtle
Genentech

Catherine Bollard
The George Washington University

Vence Bonham
National Human Genome
    Research Institute

Imein Bousnina
Genentech

Eilse Boutcher
Facing Our Risk of Cancer
    Empowered

Luke Brewster
Emory University; Atlanta Veterans
    Affairs Medical Center

Ariadne Campble
The Washington Center

Cora Trelles Cartagena
National Institutes of Health
    Vaccine Research Center

Maitreyi Chattopadhyay
Food and Drug Administration

Nimi Chhina
BioMarin Pharmaceutical Inc.

Elaine Collier
National Center for Advancing
    Translational Sciences

Kayla Cooper
National Institutes of Health

Michelle Cortes
National Institute of Dental and
    Craniofacial Research

Abla Creasey
California Institute for
    Regenerative Medicine

Sameera Daniels
Ramsey Decision Theoretics

Barto Diaz
The Consumer Goods Forum

Nancy Drakeford

Todd Durham
Foundation Fighting Blindness

Ray Ebert
National Heart, Lung, and Blood
    Institute

Sam Edland
Optum

Michael Ferenczy
GlaxoSmithKline

Tempora Fisher
National Institutes of Health

Mae Frances Frazier
U.S. Postal Service Headquarters

Dylan George
In-Q-Tel

Lawrence Goldstein
University of California, San Diego

Cynthia Golson
Department of Corrections

Mary Groesch
National Institutes of Health

Dawn Henke
Standards Coordinating Body

Brittany Hollister
National Human Genome
    Research Institute

Christopher Hug
Sanofi-Genzyme

Nina Hunter
Food and Drug Administration

Rosemarie Hunziker
Connexon Life Sciences Consulting

Jean Hu-Primmer
GlaxoSmithKline Vaccines

Ilan Irony
Food and Drug Administration

Lisa Jordan
DC/MD League for Nursing

Samira Kiani
Arizona State University

Ioannis Koutroulis
Children's National Hospital

Timothy LaVaute
National Institute of Neurological
    Disorders and Stroke, National
    Institutes of Health

Rachel Levinson
Arizona State University

Sheng Lin-Gibson
Biosystems and Biomaterials
    Division, National Institute of
    Standards and Technology

Nadya Lumelsky
National Institutes of Health

Glenn MacLean
Colorado Center for Reproductive
    Medicine

Terry Magnuson
University of North Carolina at
    Chapel Hill

Diane Maloney
Food and Drug Administration

Richard McFarland
Advanced Regenerative
    Manufacturing Institute

Paul Melmeyer
Muscular Dystrophy Association

Joseph Menetski
Foundation for the National
    Institutes of Health

Maria Millan
California Institute for
    Regenerative Medicine

Alexis Miller
Sanofi

Nancy Miller
National Cancer Institute

Jill Morris
National Institutes of Health

Jack Mosher
International Society for Stem Cell
    Research

Venkatesha Murthy
Takeda

Ramraj Singh Nayak
Guru Ghasidas University, Bilaspur
    C.G.

Lisa Neuhold
National Eye Institute

Phillip Nichols
Gwood LLC

Patrick Nosker
Affinity Asset Advisors

Kristina Obom
Johns Hopkins University

Catherine O'Riordan
Sanofi

Elizabeth Ottinger
Therapeutic Development Branch,
    National Center for Advancing
    Translational Sciences,
    National Institutes of Health

Jai Pandey
Food and Drug Administration

Bryan Parker
International Healthcare Access
    Group

Amy Patterson
National Heart, Lung, and Blood
    Institute

Duanqing Pei
Chinese Academy of Sciences

Mary Perry
National Institutes of Health

Leland Pierce
Food and Drug Administration

Anne Plant
National Institute of Standards
    and Technology

Deanna Portero
Office of Rare Diseases Research

Kimberlee Potter
Department of Veterans Affairs

Ronald Przygodzki
Department of Veterans Affairs

Yesenia Quintanilla
Prince George's County Public
    Schools

Nishadi Rajapakse
National Institutes of Health

Sesquile Ramon
Biotechnology Innovation
    Organization

Peter Reczek
Standards Coordinating Body for
    Regenerative Medicine

Barbara Redman
New York University

Derek Robertson
Maryland Sickle Cell Disease
    Association

Kelly Rose
Burroughs Wellcome Fund

Anne Rowzee
Food and Drug Administration

Krishnendu Roy
Georgia Tech; National Science
    Foundation Engineering
    Research Center for Cell
    Manufacturing Technologies

Daisy Rubio
Kaiser

Krishanu Saha
University of Wisconsin–Madison

Rachel Salzman
American Society for Gene & Cell
    Therapy

Sandhya Sanduja
Food and Drug Administration

Frank Sasinowski
Hyman, Phelps & McNamara, PC

Ivonne Schulman
National Institute of Diabetes
    and Digestive and Kidney
    Disorders

Ben Shaberman
Foundation Fighting Blindness

John Sheridan
Cystic Fibrosis Foundation

David Shindell
Odeon

Mona Shing
Food and Drug Administration

Eric Sid
National Center for Advancing
    Translational Sciences

Beth-Anne Sieber
National Institute of Neurological
    Disorders and Stroke

Jay Siegel
Food and Drug Administration;
    Johnson & Johnson (*Retired*)

Arthur Simen
Takeda

Mitchel Sivilotti
Centre for Commercialization of
    Regenerative Medicine

William Skach
Cystic Fibrosis Foundation

Lana Skirboll
Sanofi

Vivian Smith

Robert Star
National Institute of Diabetes
    and Digestive and Kidney
    Disorders

Sohel Talib
California Institute for
    Regenerative Medicine

William Tente
Humacyte

Katherine Tsokas
Johnson & Johnson

Timothy Turnham
Voz Advisors

James Valentine
Hyman, Phelps & McNamara, PC

Dan (Kelly) Wang
Food and Drug Administration

Anthony Welch
National Cancer Institute

Lis Welniak
National Heart, Lung, and Blood
    Institute

Michael Werner
Alliance for Regenerative Medicine

Keith Westby
IVERIC bio

Celia Witten
Food and Drug Administration

Ling Wong
National Institute of Neurological
    Disorders and Stroke

Cris Woolston
Sanofi

Nora Yang
Cura Ventures

Carolyn Yong
Food and Drug Administration

Lih Young

Katie Zander
Standards Coordinating Body